Snack Attack!

*Over 150 Guilt-free Treats
for Healthy Munching*

RUTH GLICK

**SMALL
STEPS
PRESS**

Director, Book Publishing, John Fedor; *Managing Editor,* Abe Ogden; *Associate Director, Consumer Books,* Robert Anthony; *Editor,* Rebecca Lanning; *Production Manager,* Melissa Sprott; *Cover Design,* Pixiedesign; *Printer,* Worzalla Publishing.

Printed in the United States of America
1 3 5 7 9 10 8 6 4 2

Small Steps Press is an imprint of the American Diabetes Association. For information about Small Steps Press or the American Diabetes Association, in English or Spanish, call 1-800-342-2383. To order other Small Steps books, call 1-800-232-6733.

Consult a health care professional before trying any of the suggestions in this publication. Small Steps Press and ADA assume no responsibility for any injury that may result from the suggestions or information in this publication.

⊗The paper in this publication meets the requirements of the ANSI Standard Z39.48-1992 (permanence of paper).

Small Steps Press titles may be purchased for business or promotional use or for special sales. To purchase more than 50 copies of this book at a discount, or for custom editions of this book with your logo, contact Lee Romano Sequeira, Special Sales & Promotions, at the address below, or at LRomano@diabetes.org or 703-299-2046.

For all other inquiries, please call 1-800-DIABETES.

Small Steps Press
1701 North Beauregard Street
Alexandria, Virginia 22311

Library of Congress Cataloging-in-Publication Data

Glick, Ruth, 1942-
   Snack attack! : guilt-free treats for healthy munching / Ruth Glick.
      p. cm.
   Includes bibliographical references and index.
   ISBN-13: 978-1-58040-228-6 (alk. paper)
   1. Low fat diet--Recipes. 2. Sugar-free diet--Recipes. 3. Snack foods. 4. Appetizers. 5. Desserts. I. Title.

   RM237.8.G59 2006
   641.5'6311--dc22

                              2006030440

Contents

Preface

Working on *Snack Attack!* has been a lot of fun for me. Creative cooking is a big part of my life, and I never stop thinking up new ideas for recipes and testing them. I particularly like coming up with dishes that can be enjoyed as mini-meals, either on my own or with friends.

In recent years, there has been a shift in thinking about good nutrition. The emphasis in the medical community used to be on lowering total fat. Now there's more recognition that the type of fat you eat is equally significant. As a result, all the recipes in this book follow these new guidelines for healthy eating.

Limiting saturated fat—from sources such as meat and dairy products—is particularly important when you're trying to eat healthfully. Even more troublesome are the hydrogenated fats (or trans fats) found in many stick margarines and commercial bakery products. But everyone loves sweets. So, as an alternative to store-bought products, try some of the easy and healthy goodies this book provides.

At the same time nutritionists were recognizing the health risks of eating trans fats, they were focusing on "good" fats—fats that can actually help to lower blood cholesterol. These are the polyunsaturated and monounsaturated fats found in oils such as canola oil and olive oil and in nuts. Also vital are the omega-3 fatty acids in oily fish such as salmon.

These new guidelines have influenced my current thinking on what to fix when I want to snack on my own or serve munchies and desserts to my friends. For example, nuts are now an important part of my plan for healthy eating, since they add both great flavor and great nutrition to many dishes. And I'm always looking for opportunities to serve fish. To add nuts to your menu, try my Peanut Butter and Marmalade Sandwich or

Pecan Pie Crust. For fish, check out my tasty Salmon Spread and Mexican Tuna Dip.

As you'll see in the recipes that follow, you can substantially expand your range of healthy treats by using Splenda, a sweetener that works well in desserts and other sweets, like my Marzipan Candy. Splenda is made from sugar, although it's very low in carbohydrates and calories. In many recipes, you can use it just the way you'd use sugar. For baking, I often use Splenda Sugar Blend, a commercial mix of sugar and Splenda with half the calories and carbohydrates of sugar. I've been very pleased with the results in recipes such as my Lemon Cheesecake and Summer Cheesecake.

You may notice that my recipes that include Splenda use a lot of vanilla extract as well. This is because many people who have tried these dishes say that Splenda can produce an aftertaste, which I've found can be counteracted with vanilla. Note that when I call for Splenda, I use the boxed product, not the packets designed for coffee and tea, since the former replaces an equal amount of sugar. However, this product is very light and tends to fly out of the measuring cup if you're not careful.

Snack Attack! includes a wide variety of recipes for you to enjoy. Some are healthier versions of old favorites, like my cheesecakes. Others are dishes I've invented, like Cranberry-Orange Tart and Tomato Soup with a Difference. The latter is definitely unusual but really good. And make sure you try some of the other exciting recipes in this book, including my Greek-Style Pizza and West African Sweet Potato–Peanut Soup.

I've had a wonderful time working on these recipes. As always, my primary goal has been to create a variety of foods that taste great, because I've followed my old, reliable philosophy that it doesn't matter how good something is for you . . . it has to be yummy if you want people to eat it.

So the next time you have a snack attack, be my guest and munch your way through these delicious and nutritious recipes—either on your own or with friends.

Acknowledgments

An enormous amount of testing went into the recipes for *Snack Attack!* I could never have accomplished all the tests and retests without Joe Galitsky, who cooked many of the recipes in my kitchen and offered suggestions for improvements in appearance, taste appeal, and flavor. I also want to thank my friends and family, especially my husband Norman Glick, my friend Binnie Braunstein, and my Thursday Writing Group, who tasted many of these dishes in their various versions and made helpful suggestions and comments.

Introduction

There's a fun side of snacking and a serious part, too. Just like meals, snacks should be nutritious, and you should remember that they are part of your daily total intake of calories, fats, carbohydrates, and proteins. All of the recipes in *Snack Attack!* follow widely recognized guidelines for healthy eating. Equally important, they're also great-tasting fare you'll want to enjoy often and serve to your friends as well. Included are more than 175 wonderful snacks, appetizers, and even desserts, designed for many different occasions—from a quick afternoon nibble to snacks that will feed a hungry crowd.

You'll find everything from creamy dips and spreads to hearty sandwiches, from chunky salads to tasty snacks. Some will feed the guys on Super Bowl Sunday. Some make great ladies' bridge club treats. Others are after-school specials that are fun for kids to make and eat. In the "Just for Kids" chapter, nutritious foods are presented in fun ways so that youngsters get used to enjoying snacks that are good for them.

All the recipes taste great. And they're an excellent way to increase the variety of beneficial foods in your diet so that healthy eating never becomes boring. Some of the recipes, like Guacamole, Nachos, Stuffed Mushrooms, and Apple Betty, are old favorites presented here in updated versions. Others are intended to expand your tastes and your definition of the snack concept. If you were raised on down-home American food, you may never have thought of fixing a Middle Eastern sandwich, eggplant sticks, or a quesadilla. Give these recipes a try. They're tasty, satisfying, and a snap to make.

You might also be surprised to find that *Snack Attack!* has a large chapter filled with flavorful salads. But if you've ever grabbed some coleslaw, potato salad, or three-bean salad out of the refrigerator for an afternoon pick-me-up, you'll understand why these dishes make great snacks. You can prepare them ahead of time and keep them for several days. And they're full of the healthy vegetables you should be eating. What's more, you don't have to worry about dressings that pile on the fat and calories. These salads are different, since they're all healthy but great-tasting alternatives to standard recipes.

One of my goals with *Snack Attack!* is to help you expand your consumption of vegetables and fruits, so I've included them in a wide variety of recipes throughout the book. In addition, vegetables star in their own chapter. And fruits are featured prominently in many of my baked goods.

Another of my goals is to keep these snacks low in fat. You'll discover that I've used a number of simple techniques for doing this. Many recipes call for judicious amounts of reduced-fat and fat-free dairy products, such as Neufchâtel cream cheese, fat-free sour cream, and reduced-fat mayonnaise. Others take advantage of reduced-fat margarine. In many recipes I use tub-style margarine that has 4.5 grams of fat per tablespoon. If you use a brand with a different fat content, the recipes might not work as well due to variations in the water content of the margarine. And tub-style margarine spreads easier than the stick variety, so you can use less. When I occasionally call for butter, it's always a small amount. But it does make a significant difference in the flavor of the finished product. In recipes calling for mayonnaise, I prefer the reduced-fat variety with 5 grams of fat per tablespoon. Often this mayonnaise is used to add a little bit of fat, and significant flavor, to salads and dips. You could use mayonnaise with less fat, but the results would not be as tasty.

In every case, I've made taste my bottom line. For example, I've been careful to boost flavor with herbs, spices, and other seasonings. Another of my standard techniques is to use a non-stick skillet where pan frying is called for. I test my culinary creations on family, friends, and colleagues and refine recipes according to their comments. Unless a dish has won praise from a broad cross-section of eaters, you won't see it here. It doesn't matter how healthy a recipe is—if it doesn't taste good and no one wants to eat it, you've wasted your time and the ingredients in making it.

You should also be aware that in conventional recipes and store-bought bakery products, sugar is often combined with ingredients that are high in fat, calories, and sodium. In *Snack Attack!* I've cut back on both fat and calories in recipes where I've used sugar. That means you can enjoy treats like Pecan Buns, Peach Cobbler, and Blueberry Muffins that are not only great tasting but also far better for you nutritionally than traditional versions.

In baked goods made from scratch, like Cranberry-Orange Muffins and Apple Scone Cake, I've increased the fiber by substituting oat bran and whole-wheat flour for some of the white flour. Another strategy I've used is to take advantage of the natural sugars in fruits, which are also high in fiber as well as vitamins and minerals.

Most of my snacks can be eaten as soon as you make them. Many will keep well in the refrigerator for several days. Where applicable, storage directions are always included. Some recipes make only enough for one or two servings but can be easily doubled. Others will feed a crowd.

There are many recipes in *Snack Attack!* that are easy and quick to make. To speed preparation time, I sometimes use the microwave for part of the cooking process, and there's even a chapter of quick, all-microwave recipes. Another tool that's very useful for creating quick snacks is the toaster oven, which I also use in a number of recipes.

Some quick dishes here use convenience foods like prepared pizza sauce, shredded reduced-fat cheese, refrigerator-case biscuits, tortillas, and stuffing mix. I appreciate convenience in the kitchen, and I use these products when I'm in a hurry.

But there's always a nutritional trade-off. And I've come to realize that the dishes I make myself, like Baked Egg Rolls, Turkey Salad, and Shrimp Remoulade, are better for my family than high-fat, high-calorie, high-sugar, high-sodium commercial preparations. Redesigning traditional recipes lets me create healthier but great-tasting versions of old favorites. Look for Better Deviled Eggs, two versions of Guacamole (one with a reduced amount of avocado and one with no avocado at all), Easy Caramel Popcorn, Mustard Pretzels, Tuna Melts, and Pecan Buns.

If you want to know the exact carbohydrate, fat, protein, and sodium content of any recipe, check its nutritional analysis, which was done by a registered dietitian. Note that if I give two alternatives in the ingredients list, such as no-salt-added tomato sauce and regular tomato sauce, the analysis is based on the first alternative. And be aware that if you make substitutions, like using reduced-fat milk instead of fat-free milk, the nutrient analysis will be different.

So the next time you have a snack attack, thumb through the pages of this book and pick something you'd like to fix. There are recipes to satisfy every taste and some that will certainly broaden your perception of the munching experience.

Spread It On

Here's a wonderful collection of tasty dips and spreads. All of them make great snacks and will keep in the refrigerator for several days after they're made. Many, like my Guacamole, Lentil Chopped Liver Spread, or Roasted Onion Spread, are also perfect for appetizers or buffet parties, where the emphasis is on grazing.

Some recipes are made primarily from high-fiber ingredients like beans and lentils. Others add fiber with celery, green onions, and sun-dried tomatoes. When I use dairy products, it's the fat-free or reduced-fat variety. Each recipe has just enough fat to give it good flavor. For example, I call for reduced-fat sour cream in my Sun-Dried Tomato Paté because it was far less tasty made with the fat-free variety. And my pestos have just enough olive oil to give them a spreadable texture.

In other recipes, I've achieved the flavor I wanted by mixing low-fat products, such as fat-free sour cream and reduced-fat mayonnaise. By the way, I use the type of reduced-calorie mayonnaise with 5 grams of fat per tablespoon, since I think it tastes close enough to the real thing to produce good results in dips, spreads, and salad dressings.

Sour Cream and Roasted Onion Spread

Roasting is a wonderful way to bring out the flavor of foods, like the onions in this simple but delicious spread. Note that the recipe calls for reduced-fat sour cream rather than the fat-free variety I use in most recipes. In this case, the change makes a significant difference in the taste of the spread.

Nonstick cooking spray

2 cups coarsely chopped onion

1 tsp olive oil

1 cup reduced-fat sour cream

2–3 drops hot pepper sauce

1/4 tsp salt (optional)

1. Preheat the oven to 400 degrees. Spray a shallow 7- by 11-inch baking pan with nonstick cooking spray. Add the onions and toss with oil.

2. Roast the onions, stirring once or twice until they are very soft and beginning to brown, about 35 to 40 minutes. Remove pan from oven and cool onions slightly.

3. Mix together the sour cream, hot pepper sauce, and salt, if desired. Stir in the onions. Serve warm or chilled on fat-free whole-wheat crackers or toasted French bread slices.

4. Cover and refrigerate leftover spread. Leftover spread will keep in the refrigerator 3 to 4 days. After refrigeration, stir before serving.

Exchanges

Free

Calories 17

Calories from Fat 9

Total Fat 1 g

Saturated Fat 0 g

Cholesterol 3 mg

Sodium 5 mg

Total Carbohydrate 2 g

Dietary Fiber 0 g

Sugars 1 g

Protein 0 g

Sun-Dried Tomato Paté

Preparation Time:
15 minutes

Serves 8

Serving Size:
2 Tbsp

This spread tastes great on half a bagel, wheat crackers, or as a stuffing for celery or Belgian endive.

1/2 cup dry-packed sun-dried tomatoes

1/4 cup water

1/2 cup reduced-fat sour cream

3 Tbsp reduced-fat mayonnaise

2 Tbsp grated Parmesan cheese

1/2 tsp basil

1 small garlic clove, chopped

1/4 cup finely chopped celery

2 Tbsp chopped chives or sliced green onion tops

1. In a 2-cup measure or similar small microwave-safe bowl, combine the tomatoes and water. Cover with wax paper and microwave on high power for 3 to 4 minutes, or until the tomatoes are softened and most of water has been absorbed. Set aside to cool for about 10 minutes.

2. Transfer to a food processor bowl and process with on-and-off bursts until the tomatoes are chopped. Transfer to a small bowl and stir in the sour cream, mayonnaise, cheese, basil, and garlic. Stir to mix well. Stir in the celery and chives. Mix well.

3. Serve at once, or cover and refrigerate. Leftover spread will keep in the refrigerator for 3 to 4 days.

Exchanges

1 Fat

Calories 50

Calories from Fat 30

Total Fat 3 g

Saturated Fat 1 g

Cholesterol 8 mg

Sodium 138 mg

Total Carbohydrate 4 g

Dietary Fiber 1 g

Sugars 1 g

Protein 1 g

Preparation Time:
  12 minutes

Serves 16

Serving Size:
  2 Tbsp

Artichoke and Shrimp Spread

Elegant but easy, this chunky dip can be served on toasted Italian bread slices or fat-free crackers.

1 13- to 14-oz can water-packed artichoke hearts, well drained
1 cup cooked small shrimp
1/4 cup fat-free sour cream
3 Tbsp reduced-fat mayonnaise
1 1/2 tsp Italian seasoning
1 garlic clove, minced
1 tsp instant minced onions
1 tsp balsamic vinegar
1/8 tsp salt, or to taste (optional)
1/8 tsp white pepper

Exchanges

1/2 Fat

Calories 26

Calories from Fat 9

Total Fat 1 g

Saturated Fat 0 g

Cholesterol 17 mg

Sodium 86 mg

Total Carbohydrate
  2 g

Dietary Fiber 0 g

Sugars 1 g

Protein 2 g

1. Remove and discard the coarse outer leaves from the artichoke hearts. Chop the hearts slightly and set them aside in a medium bowl. Chop the shrimp slightly and set them aside with the artichoke hearts.

2. In a small bowl, stir together the sour cream and mayonnaise. Add the Italian seasoning, garlic, onions, vinegar, salt (if desired), and pepper. Stir to mix well. Stir the mixture into the shrimp and artichokes.

3. Cover and refrigerate for at least 1/2 hour and up to 12 hours to allow the flavors to blend.

4. Serve on fat-free crackers or toasted Italian bread slices. Leftover spread will keep in the refrigerator for 1 to 2 days.

Cottage Cheese with Dill and Onion

Preparation Time:
12 minutes

Serves 8

Serving Size:
2 Tbsp

Use this flavored cottage cheese to stuff Belgian endive, celery, or the Dugout Canoes on page 139. For a quicker but slightly less sophisticated version of the dip, you can omit the food processor step and simply mix the ingredients together in a small bowl.

1 cup low-fat cottage cheese

1 Tbsp reduced-fat mayonnaise

2 Tbsp thinly sliced green onion tops

1/2 tsp fresh dill leaves or 1/4 tsp dried dill weed

1/8 tsp ground celery seed

Pinch of salt, or to taste (optional)

2 drops hot pepper sauce (optional)

1. Combine the cottage cheese and mayonnaise in a food processor bowl fitted with a steel blade. Process until almost smooth.

2. Turn mixture out into a small bowl. Add the onion, dill, celery seed, salt (if desired), and hot pepper sauce (if desired). Stir to mix well.

3. Serve at once, or cover and refrigerate. The dip keeps for up to 3 days in the refrigerator. Stir before serving.

Exchanges
1 Very Lean Meat

Calories 32
Calories from Fat 10
Total Fat 1 g
Saturated Fat 1 g
Cholesterol 3 mg
Sodium 125 mg
Total Carbohydrate 1 g
Dietary Fiber 0 g
Sugars 1 g
Protein 4 g

Nachos

If you love nachos but want to avoid the high-fat cheese, try this slimmed-down version. Enjoy it as a snack or serve it as an appetizer.

1 Tbsp cornstarch
1/2 tsp chili powder
1/4 tsp dry mustard
1 cup nonfat half-and-half
1 1/2 cups shredded fat-free Cheddar cheese
2/3 cup mild salsa
2 Tbsp thinly sliced green onion tops
96 regular (bite-sized) baked tortilla chips

Exchanges

1 Starch

1/2 Carbohydrate

1 Very Lean Meat

Calories 129

Calories from Fat 10

Total Fat 1 g

Saturated Fat 0.4 g

Cholesterol 4 mg

Sodium 492 mg

Total Carbohydrate
21 g

Dietary Fiber 2 g

Sugars 3 g

Protein 9 g

1. In a 4-cup measure or similar microwave-safe bowl, stir together the cornstarch, chili powder, and mustard. Add the half-and-half, stirring with a small wire whisk or fork until the cornstarch is completely incorporated. Use a spoon to make sure none of the cornstarch mixture is stuck to the bottom or sides of the bowl.

2. Cover with wax paper and microwave on high power for 2 minutes or until the mixture is very hot. Whisk with a small wire whisk. Cover and microwave again for 30 seconds on high power. Whisk. If the mixture has not thickened, repeat the heating and whisking process, 30 seconds at a time.

3. Add the cheese and stir until partially melted. Microwave the mixture for an additional 30 seconds. Then stir to completely melt the cheese. Stir in the salsa and green onion.

4. Serve warm, or cover and refrigerate for 1 to 2 days until needed. To rewarm, cover with wax paper and microwave for 1 1/2 to 2 minutes on full power. Stir.

5. To serve as a snack, lay 12 baked tortilla chips on a small plate. Pour the cheese sauce over the chips. For an appetizer, transfer to a small bowl. Guests can dip chips into the warm cheese mixture. If the mixture begins to cool, cover with wax paper and microwave for 30 to 40 seconds or keep it warm on a warming tray.

Preparation Time:
6 minutes

Serves 10

Serving Size:
1 Tbsp

Thousand Island Dressing

This tangy dressing is not only a snap to make, it's also quite versatile. Use it for dipping fresh vegetables or shrimp or as a classic salad dressing. The small amount of reduced-fat mayonnaise adds to the richness of the taste. But, if you like, you can make a completely fat-free version without the mayonnaise.

1/2 cup catsup

1/4 cup fat-free sour cream

1 Tbsp reduced-fat mayonnaise

1/2 Tbsp balsamic vinegar

1 small garlic clove, minced (optional)

1. In a small bowl, combine all the ingredients (including the garlic, if desired) and whisk together well to prevent lumps.

2. Refrigerate dressing for up to a week. After refrigeration, stir before using.

Exchanges

1 Vegetable

Calories 23

Calories from Fat 5

Total Fat 1 g

Saturated Fat 0 g

Cholesterol 1 mg

Sodium 163 mg

Total Carbohydrate 4 g

Dietary Fiber 0 g

Sugars 2 g

Protein 1 g

Guacamole

Preparation Time:
15 minutes

Serves 14

Serving Size:
2 Tbsp

If you love guacamole but hate the accompanying fat and calories, try this alternative that substitutes green peas for most of the avocado. You'll be surprised at how close this recipe comes to the taste and texture of the original.

1 1/2 cups frozen peas

1 small ripe avocado, peeled, seeded, and cut into chunks

1 Tbsp reduced-fat mayonnaise

2 tsp lemon juice

1/2 tsp cumin

1/2 tsp chili powder

1 garlic clove, minced

1/2 cup mild or medium low-sodium or regular salsa

1. In a small saucepan, combine the peas and 1/4 cup boiling water. Cover, bring to a boil, and simmer 2 minutes. Cool in a colander under cold running water. Drain well.

2. In a food processor container, combine the peas, avocado, mayonnaise, lemon juice, cumin, chili powder, and garlic. Process until blended but not absolutely smooth, stopping and scraping the container sides, if necessary. Stir in the salsa.

3. Cover and refrigerate for 1 to 2 hours or up to 24 hours to allow the flavors to blend. The dip will keep in the refrigerator for 1 to 2 days. Serve with fat-free tortilla chips.

Exchanges

1/2 Carbohydrate

Calories 32

Calories from Fat 13

Total Fat 1 g

Saturated Fat 0.2 g

Cholesterol 0 mg

Sodium 81 mg

Total Carbohydrate 4 g

Dietary Fiber 2 g

Sugars 1 g

Protein 1 g

Preparation Time:
5 minutes

Serves 12

Serving Size:
2 Tbsp

Don't Tell 'Em It's Not Guacamole

Here's a surprisingly tasty version of guacamole made with absolutely no avocado at all.

2 cups frozen peas

3 Tbsp reduced-fat mayonnaise

2 tsp lemon juice

1 tsp cumin

1/2 tsp chili powder

1 garlic clove, minced

1/2 cup mild or medium low-sodium or regular salsa

1/4 tsp salt, or to taste (optional)

1. In a small saucepan, combine the peas and 1/4 cup boiling water. Cover, bring to a boil, and simmer 2 minutes. Cool in a colander under cold running water. Drain well.

2. In a food processor container, combine the peas, mayonnaise, lemon juice, cumin, chili powder, and garlic. Process until blended but not absolutely smooth, stopping and scraping the container sides, if necessary. Stir in the salsa and salt (if desired).

3. Cover and refrigerate for 1 to 2 hours or up to 24 hours to allow flavors to blend. The mixture will keep in the refrigerator for 4 to 5 days. Serve with fat-free corn chips.

Exchanges

1/2 Starch

Calories 37

Calories from Fat 11

Total Fat 1 g

Saturated Fat 0 g

Cholesterol 2 mg

Sodium 68 mg

Total Carbohydrate
5 g

Dietary Fiber 2 g

Sugars 2 g

Protein 2 g

Salmon Salad

Preparation Time:
6 minutes

Serves 5

Serving Size:
1/4 cup

Serve this quick, tasty salad on fat-free whole-wheat crackers, on half a bagel, or on half of a whole-wheat English muffin. If you like, top with a ripe tomato slice. Or serve on a plate with lettuce, tomato, cucumbers, and any other raw vegetables you like.

1 6-oz can skinless, boneless pink salmon, well drained
1 1/2 Tbsp reduced-fat mayonnaise
1 tsp prepared white horseradish
1 large celery stalk, chopped
2 Tbsp chopped red or other sweet onion

1. Place the salmon in a small bowl. Flake to separate. Add the mayonnaise and horseradish and stir to mix well.

2. Stir in the celery and onion. Serve at once, or cover and refrigerate. Salad will keep in the refrigerator for 1 to 2 days.

Exchanges
1 Lean Meat

Calories 56

Calories from Fat 27

Total Fat 3 g

Saturated Fat 0 g

Cholesterol 17 mg

Sodium 190 mg

Total Carbohydrate
1 g

Dietary Fiber 0 g

Sugars 1 g

Protein 6 g

Tuna Salad

Preparation Time:
6 minutes

Serves 3

Serving Size:
2 Tbsp

You can serve this tasty tuna salad in a number of different ways. Spread it on a bagel half, mound it on a plate and surround it with lettuce and other vegetables, or use it to make the tuna melts on page 33.

1 3-oz can water-packed tuna, well drained
1 Tbsp reduced-fat mayonnaise
1 Tbsp chopped red bell pepper
1/2 tsp balsamic vinegar
1 Tbsp chopped chives or sliced green onion
   tops or red onion

1. In a small bowl, flake the tuna with a fork. Combine with the mayonnaise, pepper, vinegar, and chives. Stir to mix well.

2. Serve as an open-faced sandwich or as a salad surrounded by raw vegetables.

Exchanges

1 Lean Meat

Calories 48

Calories from Fat 16

Total Fat 2 g

Saturated Fat 0 g

Cholesterol 9 mg

Sodium 117 mg

Total Carbohydrate
1 g

Dietary Fiber 0 g

Sugars 0 g

Protein 7 g

Hummus with Roasted Red Peppers

Hummus is a Middle Eastern dip that is often made from ground chickpeas (garbanzo beans) and tahini (sesame butter). I prefer the milder flavor of ground sesame seeds. Roasted red peppers make a nice addition to the basic dip.

1 15-oz can chickpeas, washed and drained

1 garlic clove, minced

2 Tbsp olive oil

2 Tbsp water

1 Tbsp lemon juice

1/2 Tbsp sesame seeds

Scant 1/4 tsp salt (optional)

1/8 tsp black pepper

1/4 cup finely chopped roasted red peppers

2 Tbsp finely chopped fresh parsley

1. In a food processor container, combine the chickpeas, garlic, oil, water, lemon juice, sesame seeds, salt (if desired), and black pepper. Process until smooth. Transfer to a medium bowl.

2. Stir in the roasted peppers and parsley. If the spread seems stiff, add a bit more water. Serve at once, or cover and refrigerate for 2 to 3 hours or up to 24 hours before serving. The spread will keep in the refrigerator for 4 to 5 days. Serve with whole-wheat pita wedges or fat-free crackers.

Preparation Time: 10 minutes

Serves 12

Serving Size: 2 Tbsp

Exchanges

1/2 Starch

Calories 50

Calories from Fat 14

Total Fat 2 g

Saturated Fat 0 g

Cholesterol 0 mg

Sodium 36 mg

Total Carbohydrate 7 g

Dietary Fiber 2 g

Sugars 1 g

Protein 2 g

Serves 16

Serving Size:
2 Tbsp

Chickpea and Sun-Dried Tomato Spread

This easy spread features the wonderful combination of chickpeas (garbanzo beans) and sun-dried tomatoes. The spread can be served on fat-free crackers, whole-wheat English muffins, or pita bread wedges.

1/3 cup dry-packed sun-dried tomatoes

3 Tbsp water

1 15 1/2-oz can chickpeas, rinsed and well drained

1 8-oz can low-sodium tomato sauce or regular tomato sauce

2 Tbsp chopped chives

2 tsp olive oil

1/2 tsp Italian seasoning

1/8 tsp salt, or to taste (optional)

2–3 drops hot pepper sauce (optional)

Exchanges

1/2 Starch

Calories 42

Calories from Fat 10

Total Fat 1 g

Saturated Fat 0 g

Cholesterol 0 mg

Sodium 52 mg

Total Carbohydrate 7 g

Dietary Fiber 2 g

Sugars 1 g

Protein 2 g

1. In a small microwave-safe bowl, combine the sun-dried tomatoes and 3 Tbsp of water. Cover with wax paper and microwave on high power for 1 to 1 1/2 minutes to soften the tomatoes slightly. Drain in a colander. When the tomatoes are cool enough to handle, cut them into quarters. Set aside.

2. In a medium bowl or casserole, mash the chickpeas with a fork or potato masher until coarsely mashed. Stir in the reserved sun-dried tomatoes, tomato sauce, chives, oil, Italian seasoning, salt (if desired), and hot pepper sauce (if desired).

3. Serve at room temperature, or cover and refrigerate. Spread will keep in the refrigerator for 3 to 4 days. Stir before serving.

Lentil Chopped Liver Spread

Although this spread is made of lentils, it tastes remarkably like chopped liver.

1 1/2 cups dried brown lentils, washed and picked over
2 Tbsp instant minced onions
1 garlic clove, minced
1/3 cup liquid egg substitute
3 Tbsp reduced-fat mayonnaise
1/2 teaspoon salt, or to taste (optional)
Dash of pepper, or to taste

1. In a large saucepan, combine the lentils, onions, and garlic. Cover with 4 to 5 cups of water. Bring to a boil. Cover, reduce the heat, and simmer for 25 to 30 minutes or until lentils are tender but not mushy. Drain lentils in a colander.

2. Meanwhile, cook the egg substitute in a small nonstick skillet as if making scrambled eggs, breaking the eggs into small pieces.

3. Combine lentils and egg substitute in a medium bowl. Add the mayonnaise, salt (if desired), and pepper. Stir to mix well. Serve at once, or refrigerate for several hours before serving.

4. Serve on crackers or bagel halves. The spread will keep in the refrigerator for 3 to 4 days.

Preparation Time: 10 minutes

Serves 32

Serving Size: 2 Tbsp

Exchanges
1/2 Starch

Calories 37
Calories from Fat 5
Total Fat 1 g
Saturated Fat 0 g
Cholesterol 1 mg
Sodium 14 mg
Total Carbohydrate 5 g
Dietary Fiber 3 g
Sugars 1 g
Protein 3 g

Serves 32

Serving Size:
2 Tbsp

Herbed Lentil Spread

Lentils make delicious spreads. The only drawback is their dark brown color. If you like, garnish with chopped parsley or pimentos. This spread goes well with fat-free whole-wheat crackers. It's also wonderful on bagels or rolls.

1/2 lb brown lentils, washed and sorted
1 small onion, chopped
1 garlic clove, minced
2 Tbsp olive oil
1 1/2 Tbsp Worcestershire sauce
1 Tbsp balsamic vinegar
1 tsp Dijon-style mustard
1/4 tsp dried thyme leaves
1/4 tsp dried marjoram leaves
Generous 1/2 tsp salt, or to taste (optional)
1/8 tsp black pepper
2 celery stalks, minced

Exchanges

1/2 Starch

Calories 33

Calories from Fat 8

Total Fat 1 g

Saturated Fat 0 g

Cholesterol 0 mg

Sodium 11 mg

Total Carbohydrate 4 g

Dietary Fiber 2 g

Sugars 1 g

Protein 2 g

1. In a large pot, bring 5 cups of water to a boil. Add the lentils, onion, and garlic. Reduce the heat, cover, and simmer lentils for 35 to 45 minutes, stirring occasionally, until the lentils are very tender but not mushy. Drain in a colander.

2. Meanwhile, in a medium bowl, stir together the oil, Worcestershire sauce, vinegar, mustard, thyme, marjoram, salt (if desired), and pepper. Stir in the celery and then stir in the lentil mixture. Cover and refrigerate for 2 to 3 hours or up to 24 hours before serving. Spread will keep covered in the refrigerator for 4 to 5 days.

Tomato and Olive Tapenade

I've called for plum tomatoes in this easy, flavorful spread. However, when vine-ripened tomatoes are available in summer, feel free to use them.

5 plum tomatoes, chopped

12 large ripe pitted olives, chopped

2 Tbsp thinly sliced green onion tops

1 small garlic clove, chopped

1 tsp olive oil

2 tsp balsamic vinegar

1/4 tsp salt (optional)

1/8 tsp black pepper

1. In a medium bowl, combine the tomatoes, olives, onion, and garlic. Stir in the oil, vinegar, salt (if desired), and pepper. Transfer to a food processor container and process with 4 to 5 on-and-off bursts to further blend the vegetables. Do not overblend.

2. Serve immediately on a small slice of toasted Italian bread or whole-wheat crackers. Or cover and refrigerate for several hours and then stir before serving. Leftovers will keep in the refrigerator for 2 to 3 days.

Preparation Time: 12 minutes

Serves 22

Serving Size: 2 Tbsp

Exchanges
Free

Calories 9

Calories from Fat 5

Total Fat 1 g

Saturated Fat 0 g

Cholesterol 0 mg

Sodium 23 mg

Total Carbohydrate 1 g

Dietary Fiber 0 g

Sugars 1 g

Protein 0 g

Roasted Summer Vegetable Spread

Roasting works a magical transformation on this chunky vegetable medley. Serve warm on small slices of Italian bread or crackers. Starting the vegetables in the microwave shortens the cooking time. However, if you like, you can omit this step and roast the vegetables for about 40 to 45 minutes.

Nonstick cooking spray
4 plum tomatoes, chopped
1/2 cup diced zucchini
1/2 cup very thinly sliced onion
1/2 sweet red pepper, chopped
2 tsp olive oil
1/4 tsp dried thyme leaves
1/4 tsp salt (optional)
1/8 tsp black pepper

Exchanges

1 Vegetable

Calories 33

Calories from Fat 13

Total Fat 1 g

Saturated Fat 0 g

Cholesterol 0 mg

Sodium 5 mg

Total Carbohydrate
5 g

Dietary Fiber 1 g

Sugars 3 g

Protein 1 g

1. Preheat the oven to 400 degrees. Spray a 7- by 11-inch baking pan with nonstick cooking spray and set aside. In a medium bowl, combine the tomatoes, zucchini, onion, pepper, olive oil, thyme, salt (if desired), and black pepper. Toss to mix. Cover with wax paper and microwave for 4 to 5 minutes.

2. Transfer the vegetables to the baking pan and bake for 25 to 30 minutes, stirring occasionally, or until the onion is tender.

3. Serve at once on toasted Italian bread slices or whole-wheat crackers.

Mixed Herb Pesto

Preparation Time:
18 minutes

Serves 12

Serving Size:
1 Tbsp

If you've enjoyed pesto in Italian restaurants, you may be surprised by how easy it is to make at home. This recipe is not only flavorful, it's also lower in fat than traditional versions.

2 Tbsp pine nuts

3 garlic cloves

1 1/4 cups packed fresh basil leaves

1/4 cup packed chopped fresh chives or green onions

1/4 cup packed fresh parsley leaves

3 Tbsp freshly grated Parmesan cheese

1 Tbsp fresh lemon juice

Generous 1/4 teaspoon salt or more, to taste

3 Tbsp extra virgin olive oil

1. Spread the pine nuts in a small, nonstick skillet. Cook over medium-high heat, stirring constantly, until the nuts begin to turn brown and smell toasted, about 3 to 4 minutes. Immediately transfer to a plate and cool slightly.

2. Combine the nuts, garlic, basil, chives, parsley, cheese, lemon juice, and salt in a food processor. Process until finely minced. With the processor on, slowly pour the oil through the food tube; process until well blended, stopping and scraping down the sides of the container once or twice.

3. Transfer to a small bowl. Serve at room temperature, or cover with a tight seal and refrigerate. Pesto will keep in the refrigerator for 2 to 3 days.

Exchanges

1 Fat

Calories 49

Calories from Fat 42

Total Fat 5 g

Saturated Fat 1 g

Cholesterol 1 mg

Sodium 73 mg

Total Carbohydrate 1 g

Dietary Fiber 0 g

Sugars 1 g

Protein 1 g

Sun-Dried Tomato Pesto

Preparation Time:
18 minutes

Serves 18

Serving Size:
1 Tbsp

Sun-dried tomatoes give this easy pesto a distinctive tang. Serve it on crostini (toasted Italian bread slices) or fat-free crackers.

1 cup dry-packed sun-dried tomatoes

1/4 cup water

1 cup packed fresh basil leaves

1/3 cup chopped chives

1/4 cup fat-free Parmesan cheese topping

3 Tbsp extra virgin olive oil

2 garlic cloves, minced

1/8 tsp black pepper

1. In a 2-cup measure or similar small microwave-safe bowl, combine the sun-dried tomatoes and water. Cover with wax paper and microwave on high power for 2 minutes or until the tomatoes are slightly softened.

2. In a food processor bowl, process the tomatoes and water until the tomatoes are coarsely chopped. Remove to a small bowl and set aside. In the food processor bowl, combine the basil, chives, Parmesan cheese, oil, garlic, and pepper. Process until chopped.

3. Stir the basil mixture into the tomatoes. Serve at room temperature, or cover and refrigerate until serving. The pesto will keep for 2 to 3 days in the refrigerator.

Exchanges

1/2 Fat

Calories 36

Calories from Fat 21

Total Fat 2 g

Saturated Fat 1 g

Cholesterol 0 mg

Sodium 87 mg

Total Carbohydrate 3 g

Dietary Fiber 0 g

Sugars 1 g

Protein 1 g

Sandwich Board

The recipes in this chapter are for sandwiches you can make quickly and eat at once. Most make one or two servings, although a few are designed to feed a crowd. Many, like my Grilled Portobello Mushroom Sandwich and Falafel, are designed to expand your concept of a sandwich.

Some are presented open-faced on a slice of whole-wheat bread. Others are made on half an English muffin, stuffed into a pita pocket, or rolled in a tortilla. If you like, double the recipe and make it for lunch instead of a snack. Or try the Egg 'n' Muffin recipes for breakfast.

When possible, make your sandwiches with whole-wheat, mixed grain, or oat bran bread rather than plain white or wheat bread, since this is an easy way to add fiber to your diet.

Egg 'n' Muffin

Preparation Time:
6 minutes

Serves 2

Serving Size:
1 muffin half

This spicy egg and muffin sandwich is great for breakfast, lunch, or a snack any time. For crunch, you can also add a little chopped celery to the egg substitute before cooking.

Nonstick cooking spray

1/2 cup frozen mixed pepper and onion stir-fry

1/3 cup liquid egg substitute

Pinch dry mustard

Pinch black pepper

1 Tbsp catsup

1 whole-wheat or oat bran English muffin, split in half

2 Tbsp reduced-fat shredded Cheddar cheese

1. In a medium nonstick skillet coated with nonstick spray, cook the pepper and onion mixture over medium-high heat until the onion is tender, 2 or 3 minutes.

2. Lower the heat to medium. Add the egg substitute and mustard and cook, stirring occasionally, until the egg is cooked through, about 2 minutes. Remove from heat and stir in catsup.

3. Spread the mixture evenly on open, untoasted English muffin halves. Sprinkle with cheese. Toast in toaster oven or under broiler until cheese is just melted and muffins are warmed.

Exchanges

1 Starch

1 Very Lean Meat

Calories 123

Calories from Fat 21

Total Fat 2 g

Saturated Fat 1 g

Cholesterol 5 mg

Sodium 333 mg

Total Carbohydrate 17 g

Dietary Fiber 2 g

Sugars 5 g

Protein 10 g

Egg 'n' Muffin, Mexican Style

Here's a spicy variation of my basic Egg 'n' Muffin sandwich.

Nonstick cooking spray
1/3 cup liquid egg substitute
1/4 tsp chili powder
1/8 tsp salt (optional)
3 Tbsp mild or medium salsa
1 whole-wheat English muffin, split in half
2 Tbsp reduced-fat shredded Cheddar or Jack cheese

1. In a medium-sized nonstick skillet coated with nonstick spray, stir together the egg substitute, chili powder, and salt (if desired). Cook over medium heat, stirring occasionally, until cooked through, about 2 minutes. Remove from heat and stir in salsa.

2. Spread the mixture evenly on open, untoasted English muffin halves. Sprinkle with cheese. Toast in toaster oven or under broiler until cheese is just melted and muffins are warmed.

Preparation Time:
6 minutes

Serves 2

Serving Size:
1 muffin half

Exchanges
1 Starch
1 Very Lean Meat

Calories 115
Calories from Fat 21
Total Fat 2 g
Saturated Fat 1 g
Cholesterol 5 mg
Sodium 307 mg
Total Carbohydrate 15 g
Dietary Fiber 2 g
Sugars 3 g
Protein 10 g

Serves 2

Serving Size:
1 muffin half

Egg 'n' Muffin, Italian Style

Here's an Italian-style variation of my basic Egg 'n' Muffin sandwich.

Nonstick cooking spray
1/3 cup liquid egg substitute
1 Tbsp thinly sliced green onion tops
1/4 tsp Italian seasoning
1 whole-wheat English muffin, split in half
1 Tbsp grated Parmesan cheese
2 thin slices fresh tomato
Chopped parsley for garnish (optional)

1. In a medium-sized nonstick skillet coated with nonstick spray coating, stir together the egg substitute, green onion, and Italian seasoning. Cook over medium heat, stirring occasionally, until cooked through, about 2 minutes.

2. Remove from heat and spread the mixture evenly on open, untoasted English muffin halves. Sprinkle with cheese and top with tomato.

3. Toast in toaster oven or under the broiler until the cheese is just melted and muffins are warmed. If desired, sprinkle with chopped parsley.

Exchanges

1 Starch

1 Very Lean Meat

Calories 106

Calories from Fat 17

Total Fat 2 g

Saturated Fat 1 g

Cholesterol 4 mg

Sodium 248 mg

Total Carbohydrate
15 g

Dietary Fiber 2 g

Sugars 3 g

Protein 9 g

Grilled Portobello Mushroom Sandwich

Try this extremely versatile recipe for a grilled portobello mushroom sandwich. You can garnish your sandwich with a little balsamic vinegar, Dijon-style mustard, or a few drops of hot pepper sauce. You can also grill a tomato slice along with the mushroom and add onions, sprouts, or field greens.

1 portobello mushroom
Desired vegetables (optional)
1/2 toasted English muffin or other bread
Pinch salt
Pinch black pepper

1. Preheat the broiler. Place the mushroom and any vegetables you wish to grill on a small baking sheet. Broil 2 inches from the heat for about 3 minutes on each side or until the mushroom has shrunk slightly, exuded its juice, and begun to brown.

2. Serve on a toasted English muffin half, sprinkle with salt and pepper, and garnish as desired.

Preparation Time: 2 minutes

Serves 1

Serving Size: 1 muffin half

Exchanges
1 Starch
1 Vegetable

Calories 94
Calories from Fat 9
Total Fat 1 g
Saturated Fat 0 g
Cholesterol 0 mg
Sodium 136 mg
Total Carbohydrate 18 g
Dietary Fiber 2 g
Sugars 3 g
Protein 4 g

Quick Fajitas

With this quick-as-a-wink recipe, you can easily create restaurant-style fajitas at home. If you want to double or triple the recipe, use a larger skillet.

Nonstick cooking spray
1/2 cup frozen mixed pepper and onion stir-fry
1 oz cooked diced turkey breast meat or shrimp
1 6-inch low-fat flour tortilla
1–2 Tbsp mild or medium salsa

1. Coat a medium nonstick skillet with nonstick spray. Add the pepper and onion mixture and turkey or shrimp and cook over medium-high heat, stirring frequently, until the onions are softened, about 2 minutes.

2. Place the tortilla on a small plate. Spoon the pepper mixture over the tortilla. Add the salsa. Place the tortilla in the pan and reduce the heat to medium-low. Cover the skillet and cook for 1 minute, until the tortilla is heated.

3. Fold the tortilla in half and serve.

Exchanges

1 Starch

1 Vegetable

1 Very Lean Meat

Calories 126

Calories from Fat 3

Total Fat 0 g

Saturated Fat 0 g

Cholesterol 23 mg

Sodium 303 mg

Total Carbohydrate 20 g

Dietary Fiber 2 g

Sugars 2 g

Protein 12 g

Middle Eastern Sandwich

Capture the flavors of the Middle East in this quick and tasty sandwich.

Nonstick cooking spray
1/2 cup frozen mixed pepper and onion stir-fry
3 Tbsp chopped fresh tomato
1 Tbsp dark raisins
1 garlic clove, minced
Pinch dried thyme leaves
Pinch cinnamon
1 small whole-wheat pita bread, cut in half

1. In a medium nonstick skillet coated with non-stick spray, combine the pepper-onion mixture, tomato, raisins, garlic, thyme, and cinnamon. Stir to mix well. Cook over medium heat, stirring occasionally with a wooden spoon, until the onions are softened, about 2 to 3 minutes.

2. Divide mixture evenly in pita pockets and serve.

Preparation Time:
5 minutes

Serves 2

Serving Size:
1 pita bread half

Exchanges

1 Starch

1 Vegetable

Calories 96

Calories from Fat 7

Total Fat 1 g

Saturated Fat 0 g

Cholesterol 0 mg

Sodium 71 mg

Total Carbohydrate 21 g

Dietary Fiber 2 g

Sugars 6 g

Protein 3 g

Preparation Time:
20 minutes

Serves 11

Serving Size:
1 Tbsp and
1/2 oz bread

Exchanges

1 Starch

1/2 Fat

Calories 104

Calories from Fat 21

Total Fat 2 g

Saturated Fat 0 g

Cholesterol 0 mg

Sodium 118 mg

Total Carbohydrate
17 g

Dietary Fiber 3 g

Sugars 3 g

Protein 4 g

Imported from the Middle East, falafel is a patty made of chickpeas and sesame butter and is traditionally deep-fried. However, I like it even better in this baked version.

1 15-oz can chickpeas (garbanzo beans), rinsed and drained
2 Tbsp tahini (sesame butter)
2 Tbsp liquid egg substitute
2 Tbsp minced green onion tops
2 garlic cloves, minced
1 tsp cumin
1/2 tsp turmeric
1/4 tsp salt, or to taste (optional)
1/8 tsp black pepper
Nonstick cooking spray
1 small onion, chopped
1 medium tomato, chopped
1/2 cup shredded lettuce
1 small cucumber, seeded and chopped
Pita pockets, cut into halves or wedges

1. Preheat the oven to 400 degrees. In a food processor container fitted with a steel blade, process the chickpeas until ground, stopping and scraping down sides of the container if necessary. (Or mash by hand.)

2. Transfer to a medium bowl and add the tahini, egg substitute, green onion, garlic, cumin, turmeric, salt (if desired), and pepper. Stir to mix well.

3. Spray a large baking sheet with nonstick cooking spray. Drop mixture by rounded tablespoon-
fuls onto baking sheet, flattening each portion
and shaping into a patty with fingers. Bake on
the center oven rack for 5 minutes. Turn with a
spatula. Bake for an additional 4 to 5 minutes
until cooked through.

4. Serve in pita pockets with onion, tomato,
lettuce, and cucumber. Falafel will keep in the
refrigerator for 2 to 3 days and can be reheated
quickly in the microwave or in a toaster oven on
a small sheet of aluminum foil. They can also be
frozen on a cookie sheet, transferred to a plastic
bag, and kept in the freezer for several weeks.

Eggplant Mini-Pita Pocket Sandwiches

These vegetarian mini-pita sandwiches make a particularly nice warm-weather snack.

Nonstick cooking spray

1 medium (about 1 lb) eggplant, halved lengthwise

1 medium onion, peeled, halved, and lightly rubbed with olive oil

2 medium garlic cloves, peeled and minced

1/4 cup finely minced parsley

1/4 cup plain fat-free yogurt

1/4 tsp salt, or to taste (optional)

1/4 tsp black pepper, or to taste

1 Tbsp olive oil

1–2 tsp fresh lemon juice, or to taste

6 mini onion-flavored or plain pita pockets (4-inch diameter)

1/4 cup each coarsely chopped tomato and peeled cucumber, mixed

Exchanges

1 Starch

2 Vegetable

1/2 Fat

Calories 140

Calories from Fat 27

Total Fat 3 g

Saturated Fat 1 g

Cholesterol 0 mg

Sodium 173 mg

Total Carbohydrate 25 g

Dietary Fiber 3 g

Sugars 6 g

Protein 4 g

1. Preheat the oven to 450 degrees. Line a large rimmed baking sheet with foil. Lightly spray the foil with nonstick cooking spray.

2. Lay the eggplant and onion cut-side down on the foil. Roast for 20 to 25 minutes, or until the eggplant halves are just tender when pierced with a fork.

3. Let the vegetables stand until cool enough to handle. Remove the skin from the eggplant. Chop the eggplant and onion fine enough to form a rough puree.

4. Turn out into a bowl. Stir in the garlic, parsley, yogurt, salt (if desired), pepper, oil, and lemon juice. Cover and refrigerate for at least 1/2 hour or up to 3 to 4 days, if desired.

5. To serve, stuff a pocket with eggplant filling and then top with a generous tablespoon of tomato-cucumber mixture. Recipe makes enough filling for 6 mini pita pockets. Leftover filling and tomato-cucumber mixture can be covered and refrigerated for 2 to 3 days.

Pepper and Onion Quesadilla

Vegetables add crunch and taste appeal to this quesadilla.

Nonstick cooking spray

1/2 cup frozen mixed pepper and onion stir-fry

1 6-inch thin low-fat flour tortilla (0.5 gram of fat or less per tortilla)

1/4 cup shredded fat-free Cheddar cheese (1 oz)

1–2 Tbsp mild or medium salsa (optional)

1. Coat a medium nonstick skillet with nonstick cooking spray. Add the pepper and onion mixture and cook over medium-high heat, stirring frequently, until the onions are softened, about 2 minutes.

2. Push the pepper and onion mixture to the side of the pan. Add the tortilla. Scoop up the pepper and onion mixture and arrange it evenly over the tortilla. Sprinkle with the cheese. Reduce the heat to medium low. Cover the skillet and cook until the cheese is melted, 2 to 3 minutes.

3. If desired, spoon salsa over the melted cheese. Fold the tortilla and serve.

Exchanges

1 Starch

1 Vegetable

1 Very Lean Meat

Calories 125

Calories from Fat 1

Total Fat 0 g

Saturated Fat 0 g

Cholesterol 3 mg

Sodium 499 mg

Total Carbohydrate 20 g

Dietary Fiber 2 g

Sugars 2 g

Protein 12 g

Tuna Melts

Preparation Time:
 8 minutes

Serves 3

Serving Size:
 1 tuna melt

This tasty tuna melt starts with the easy tuna salad on page 12.

1 recipe tuna salad (p. 12)
3 Tbsp grated sharp Cheddar cheese
3 whole-wheat or oat bran English muffin halves

1. Divide the tuna salad equally among the English muffin halves, spreading it out over the muffin surface.

2. Sprinkle the cheese on top of the tuna mixture, dividing evenly. Toast until cheese is melted.

Exchanges
1 Starch
1 Lean Meat

Calories 130
Calories from Fat 36
Total Fat 4 g
Saturated Fat 1 g
Cholesterol 14 mg
Sodium 256 mg
Total Carbohydrate 14 g
Dietary Fiber 2 g
Sugars 2 g
Protein 10 g

Serves 1

Serving Size:
1 wrap

Turkey and Tomato Wrap

A little turkey goes a long way in this quick wrap. And fresh basil really does make a difference in the taste. If it's unavailable, you could substitute dried basil.

1 6-inch low-fat flour tortilla

2 tsp reduced-fat mayonnaise

2 slices deli-style fat-free roasted turkey breast

2 Tbsp chopped fresh tomato

1 Tbsp chopped fresh basil leaves (or 1/8 tsp dried basil)

1. Lay the tortilla flat on a small plate. Spread with the mayonnaise. Lay the turkey slices on the tortilla. Sprinkle the tortilla with the tomato and basil.

2. Roll the tortilla and turkey around the tomato-basil filling. Eat like a rolled sandwich.

Exchanges

1 Starch

1 Lean Meat

Calories 147

Calories from Fat 30

Total Fat 3 g

Saturated Fat 1 g

Cholesterol 27 mg

Sodium 297 mg

Total Carbohydrate 19 g

Dietary Fiber 1 g

Sugars 1 g

Protein 12 g

Vegetable Wrap

Preparation Time:
5 minutes

Serves 2

Serving Size:
1 wrap

You can make the vegetable mixture, serve half of it in a tortilla, and save the rest in the refrigerator for the next day. If you like, substitute large lettuce or romaine leaves for the tortillas.

1/2 cup peeled, chopped cucumber
1/4 cup chopped sweet red or green pepper
2 large pitted black olives, chopped
1 large plum tomato, chopped
2 Tbsp thinly sliced green onion tops
1/4 cup reduced-fat sour cream
1/2 tsp Italian seasoning
2 small low-fat flour tortillas

1. In a small bowl, combine the cucumber, pepper, olives, tomato, and green onion. Stir to mix. Stir in the sour cream and the Italian seasoning.

2. Divide the filling evenly between the two flour tortillas, laying the mixture in a line down the center of each. Roll each tortilla around the filling. Serve immediately.

Exchanges

1 Starch

1 Vegetable

1 Fat

Calories 161

Calories from Fat 48

Total Fat 5 g

Saturated Fat 1 g

Cholesterol 10 mg

Sodium 211 mg

Total Carbohydrate 24 g

Dietary Fiber 3 g

Sugars 5 g

Protein 4 g

Pan-Grilled Vegetable Wrap

I've used a little olive oil in this recipe because it helps cook the vegetables and improves their texture. If you'd like, you can substitute nonstick cooking spray. However, the vegetables will take longer to cook.

2 tsp olive oil
1 cup frozen mixed pepper and onion stir-fry
3/4 cup chopped broccoli or cauliflower florets
1/2 cup chopped zucchini
1 garlic clove, minced
Generous 1/2 tsp Italian seasoning
1/8 tsp salt (optional)
Pinch black pepper
2 small low-fat flour tortillas

Exchanges

1 Starch

1 Vegetable

1 Fat

Calories 170

Calories from Fat 64

Total Fat 7 g

Saturated Fat 1 g

Cholesterol 0 mg

Sodium 169 mg

Total Carbohydrate
23 g

Dietary Fiber 3 g

Sugars 4 g

Protein 5 g

1. Place the olive oil in a medium nonstick skillet. Add the onion and pepper mixture, broccoli, zucchini, garlic, Italian seasoning, salt (if desired), and pepper. Cook over medium-high heat, stirring frequently, until the vegetables are tender-crisp and begin to brown slightly, about 4 to 5 minutes.

2. To warm the tortillas, transfer the vegetables to a small plate. Lower the heat and place each tortilla, one at a time, in the skillet for 30 to 40 seconds.

3. Divide the vegetables between the tortillas, wrapping the tortilla around the filling. Serve immediately.

South of the Border Pizza

Say olé to this easy pizza variation made with salsa and Cheddar cheese and served on an English muffin half.

Nonstick cooking spray

1/3 cup frozen mixed pepper and onion stir-fry

Scant 1/4 cup mild or medium salsa

1 whole-wheat English muffin, separated into halves

1/3 cup shredded fat-free Cheddar cheese

1. In a medium nonstick skillet coated with nonstick cooking spray, cook the onion and pepper mixture over medium heat, stirring frequently, until the onion is tender, about 4 to 6 minutes.

2. Meanwhile, divide the salsa evenly between the English muffin halves and spread it evenly over each half. Sprinkle the cheese evenly over the two halves. Toast the muffin halves in a toaster oven or under the broiler until the cheese melts.

3. When the vegetable mixture is cooked, spread it evenly over the pizzas.

Preparation Time:
3 minutes

Serves 2

Serving Size:
1 muffin half plus topping

Exchanges

1 Starch

1 Very Lean Meat

Calories 104

Calories from Fat 7

Total Fat 1 g

Saturated Fat 0 g

Cholesterol 2 mg

Sodium 487 mg

Total Carbohydrate 17 g

Dietary Fiber 2 g

Sugars 4 g

Protein 9 g

Serves 1

Serving Size:
1 open-faced
sandwich

Egg Salad Sandwich

You've probably used fat-free egg substitute (which is made from egg whites) in cooked dishes. But here's another idea. If you love egg salad but have cut it from your meal plan because of the cholesterol, try this zippy recipe. With all the taste of traditional egg salad and far less fat, it's one of my favorite sandwiches.

1/4 cup fat-free egg substitute

2 tsp reduced-fat mayonnaise

1 tsp sweet or unsweetened pickle relish

1/8 tsp Dijon mustard

Pinch salt (optional)

1 Tbsp finely chopped celery

1 slice regular or low-carb whole-wheat bread,
    untoasted or toasted

Exchanges

1 Starch

1 Very Lean Meat

1/2 Fat

1. In a small, nonstick skillet over medium to medium-low heat, cook and scramble the egg substitute. Transfer to a small bowl and cool slightly.

2. Add the mayonnaise, pickle relish, mustard, and salt, if desired. Add the celery and stir to mix well.

3. Spread on a slice of the bread. Serve as an open-faced sandwich.

Calories 137

Calories from Fat 39

Total Fat 4 g

Saturated Fat 0.7 g

Cholesterol 3 mg

Sodium 404 mg

Total Carbohydrate
17 g

Dietary Fiber 2 g

Sugars 4 g

Protein 9 g

Quick Turkey Salad Sandwich

Roasted turkey breast is wonderfully low in fat but high in flavor. Here it's spiced up with red onion and balsamic vinegar. Instead of serving the turkey salad on an English muffin half, you could roll it in a flour tortilla.

3/4 oz roasted turkey breast

1 Tbsp fat-free sour cream

1 tsp reduced-fat mayonnaise

1/2 Tbsp chopped red onion

1/4 tsp balsamic vinegar

Pinch of salt and pepper

Pinch of dried rosemary leaves, or
    1/4 tsp fresh rosemary

1/2 oat bran English muffin, toasted

1. Cut the turkey into very small bite-sized pieces. Set aside.

2. In a small bowl, stir together the sour cream, mayonnaise, onion, vinegar, salt, pepper, and rosemary. Stir in the turkey.

3. Mound the mixture on an English muffin half.

Preparation Time:
5 minutes

Serves 1

Serving Size:
1 muffin half

Exchanges

1 Starch

1 Very Lean Meat

Calories 123

Calories from Fat 21

Total Fat 2 g

Saturated Fat 0 g

Cholesterol 19 mg

Sodium 181 mg

Total Carbohydrate
16 g

Dietary Fiber 2 g

Sugars 4 g

Protein 10 g

Just for Fun

Here are some recipes I wanted to include in *Snack Attack!* but simply couldn't classify under any other heading. Included are a number of real treats, such as Better Deviled Eggs, that go a long way toward reducing the fat and cholesterol in traditional snack and picnic favorites.

Two recipes, Parmesan Triangles and Asian Triangles, are made with wonton wrappers, which are sold in the produce department of most large supermarkets. They're fat free and crisp up nicely when garnished and baked in the oven.

Pico de Gallo

Preparation Time:
20 minutes

Serves 20

Serving Size:
2 Tbsp

Pico de gallo is simply the Spanish name for fresh salsa. The name means "rooster's beak" because salsa can have quite a bite, depending on the chilis used. In summer, I make this dip with ripe tomatoes. In winter, I use plum tomatoes. If you dislike the distinctive taste of cilantro, you can leave it out. Be sure to wash your hands thoroughly after handling hot chili peppers, as they can leave an oily residue on your skin that can irritate your eyes.

2 fresh, mild jalapeño chili peppers, seeds and membranes removed, finely chopped

2 cups diced fresh tomatoes

1/2 cup thinly sliced green onions, white and green parts

2 Tbsp chopped cilantro

Grated zest of 1 lime

1–2 Tbsp fresh lime juice, or to taste

1/4 tsp salt, or to taste (optional)

Exchanges
Free

1. In a medium bowl, combine the chilis, tomatoes, onions, cilantro, lime zest, lime juice, and salt (if desired). Stir to mix well.

2. Serve immediately with fat-free tortilla chips, or cover and refrigerate for 3 to 4 hours before serving. Pico de gallo will keep in the refrigerator for 3 to 4 days.

Calories 7

Calories from Fat 1

Total Fat 0 g

Saturated Fat 0 g

Cholesterol 0 mg

Sodium 2 mg

Total Carbohydrate 2 g

Dietary Fiber 0 g

Sugars 1 g

Protein 0 g

Preparation Time:
15 minutes

Serves 28

Serving Size:
2 Tbsp

Black Bean Salsa

Serve this fresh and spicy salsa with fat-free tortilla chips. Be sure to wash your hands well after handling hot chili peppers, since the oily residue left on your skin can cause eye irritation.

1 large tomato, chopped

1/4 cup thinly sliced green onion tops

1/2 sweet red or green pepper, seeded and chopped

1 medium jalapeño chili pepper, seeds and membrane removed, chopped

2 tsp olive oil

2 tsp lemon juice

1/4 tsp dried oregano leaves

1 large garlic clove, minced

1/4 tsp salt, or to taste (optional)

1 3/4 cups cooked black beans, or 1 15-oz can black beans, rinsed and well drained

Exchanges

Free

Calories 20

Calories from Fat 4

Total Fat 0 g

Saturated Fat 0 g

Cholesterol 0 mg

Sodium 1 mg

Total Carbohydrate
3 g

Dietary Fiber 1 g

Sugars 1 g

Protein 1 g

1. In a medium bowl, combine the tomato, green onions, sweet pepper, chili pepper, olive oil, lemon juice, oregano, garlic, and salt (if desired). Stir to mix well.

2. Carefully stir in the black beans. Serve at once, or cover and refrigerate for 1 hour or up to 24 hours before serving.

3. The salsa will keep for 4 to 5 days in the refrigerator. Serve with fat-free tortilla chips.

Better Deviled Eggs

Preparation Time:
3 minutes

Serves 2

Serving Size:
1 egg

This is a healthier version of a traditional favorite.

2 hard-cooked large eggs, cooled under running water

2 tsp fat-free sour cream

1 tsp sweet pickle relish

1 tsp reduced-fat mayonnaise

1/8–1/4 tsp Dijon-style mustard

Pinch salt (optional)

2 Tbsp finely chopped celery

1. Cut each egg in half. Carefully remove the yolks. Discard one yolk.

2. In a custard cup, mash the remaining egg yolk. Add the sour cream, pickle relish, mayonnaise, mustard, and salt (if desired). Stir to mix well. Stir in the celery.

3. Serve at once, or cover and refrigerate. Deviled eggs will keep in the refrigerator for 1 to 2 days.

Exchanges

1 Lean Meat

Calories 64

Calories from Fat 30

Total Fat 3 g

Saturated Fat 1 g

Cholesterol 107 mg

Sodium 121 mg

Total Carbohydrate 3 g

Dietary Fiber 0 g

Sugars 2 g

Protein 5 g

Easy Corn Relish

Preparation Time:
15 minutes

Serves 16

Serving Size:
2 Tbsp

Serve this corn relish on fat-free crackers or on a whole-wheat or oat bran English muffin half.

2 cups frozen corn kernels, cooked according to package directions

2/3 cup chili sauce

1 celery stalk, chopped

1/2 red bell pepper, seeded and chopped

2 Tbsp chopped chives or thinly sliced green onion tops

1 tsp olive oil

1/4 tsp dried thyme leaves

1 garlic clove, minced

1. Cool the cooked corn in a colander under cold running water. Drain.

2. In a medium bowl, combine the chili sauce, celery, red pepper, chives, oil, thyme, and garlic. Stir to mix well. Stir in the corn.

3. Serve at room temperature, or cover and refrigerate. Relish will keep in the refrigerator for 3 to 4 days.

Exchanges

1/2 Starch

Calories 32

Calories from Fat 4

Total Fat 0 g

Saturated Fat 0 g

Cholesterol 0 mg

Sodium 138 mg

Total Carbohydrate 7 g

Dietary Fiber 1 g

Sugars 2 g

Protein 1 g

Strawberry-Peach Cooler

This easy, refreshing fruit shake has become one of my summer favorites. I love the natural tartness of the fruit combination, but if you'd prefer a sweeter drink, add a small amount of artificial sweetener to taste. The partially frozen fruit gives the shake its icy texture.

1 cup dry-packed unsweetened frozen straw-
    berries
2/3 cup dry-packed unsweetened frozen
    peaches
3/4 cup orange juice

1. In a 2-cup measure or similar microwave-safe bowl, combine the strawberries and peaches. Cover with wax paper and microwave on high power for 45 seconds to 1 minute to thaw the fruit slightly. The fruit should be icy but not hard. Working with a small knife in the measuring cup, cut each peach slice in half.

2. Transfer the peaches and strawberries to a blender container. Add the orange juice. Blend on low power to combine. Then increase power to high and continue to blend until the peaches are completely pureed, at least 1 1/2 minutes.

Exchanges

2 Fruit

Calories 105

Calories from Fat 2

Total Fat 0 g

Saturated Fat 0 g

Cholesterol 0 mg

Sodium 2 mg

Total Carbohydrate
26 g

Dietary Fiber 3 g

Sugars 23 g

Protein 2 g

Serves 2

Serving Size:
1 generous cup

Mango Lassi

Lassi, a tart, cooling yogurt drink, is a treat I've learned to enjoy in Indian restaurants. Happily, it's easy to make at home. Mango is one of the traditional fruit flavors used.

1 ripe mango
1 8-oz carton reduced-fat yogurt
1/2 cup very cold water

1. Remove the flesh from the mango, discarding the skin and seed. You should have about 1 cup of mango.

2. Combine the mango, yogurt, and water in a blender container. Blend on medium speed until well combined and smooth. Serve at once.

3. Leftover lassi can be tightly covered and kept in the refrigerator for 24 hours. Stir before serving.

Exchanges

1 Fruit

1/2 Reduced-Fat
Milk

Calories 128

Calories from Fat 20

Total Fat 2 g

Saturated Fat 1 g

Cholesterol 10 mg

Sodium 88 mg

Total Carbohydrate
23 g

Dietary Fiber 2 g

Sugars 21 g

Protein 7 g

Banana-Strawberry Shake

Be sure to use a very ripe banana in this tart and refreshing fruit shake.

1 small very ripe banana, cut into large chunks
1 cup dry-packed unsweetened frozen strawberries
1 cup low-fat (1%) milk

In a blender container, combine the banana, strawberries, and milk. Blend on medium speed until the strawberries are completely pureed and the shake is smooth. Serve at once.

Preparation Time:
4 minutes

Serves 2

Serving Size:
1 1/4 cups

Exchanges
1 Fruit
1/2 Fat-Free Milk

Calories 117
Calories from Fat 14
Total Fat 2 g
Saturated Fat 1 g
Cholesterol 5 mg
Sodium 64 mg
Total Carbohydrate 23 g
Dietary Fiber 3 g
Sugars 17 g
Protein 5 g

Screws and Bolts

I fell in love with this homemade snack mix the first time I tasted it at a friend's house after school. For me, it was an exotic treat, since my mother bought all of her crunchy snacks from the grocery store. This version retains the intense flavor of the original.

Nonstick cooking spray

1/4 cup reduced-fat tub-style margarine (4.5 g fat/T)

2 Tbsp Worcestershire sauce

1 tsp chili powder

1 tsp paprika

Pinch garlic powder

1/2 tsp salt, or to taste (optional)

3–4 drops hot pepper sauce

3 cups unsalted thin pretzels (large pieces broken up before measuring)

2 cups wheat squares cereal

2 cups bran squares cereal

1 cup toasted oat O's cereal

1/2 cup raisins

1/2 cup chopped dried apricots

1. Preheat the oven to 300 degrees. Coat a large, shallow baking pan with nonstick cooking spray and set aside.

2. In a 1-cup measure or similar small microwave-safe bowl, mix together the margarine, Worcestershire sauce, chili powder, paprika, garlic powder, salt (if desired), and hot pepper sauce. Cover with wax paper and microwave on high

power for about 1 minute or until the margarine is almost melted. Stir to combine ingredients. Set aside.

3. In the baking pan, combine the pretzels, wheat squares, bran squares, and toasted oat O's. Slowly drizzle the margarine mixture over the cereal mixture, lifting and stirring very well to coat the cereal and pretzels as evenly as possible.

4. Bake for 25 minutes, stirring twice to prevent mixture on the bottom from burning, or until mixture is crisp. Cool the pan on a wire rack. Stir in the raisins and apricots while the mixture is still warm.

5. Cool before serving. Store in an airtight container. The mixture will keep for up to a week at room temperature.

Serves 10

Serving Size:
1 cup

Easy Cheese Popcorn

Popcorn makes a great snack. Here's a cheese popcorn that won't bust your fat budget.

10 cups air-popped or low-fat microwave
    popcorn
3 oz (about 3/4 cup) shredded reduced-fat
    Cheddar cheese

1. Preheat the oven to 375 degrees. Remove any unpopped kernels from the popcorn, and spread the popcorn on a large cookie sheet with sides. Popcorn should cover the pan bottom in a single layer, with as few as possible spaces in between kernels.

Exchanges

1/2 Starch

1/2 Fat

2. Slowly sprinkle the cheese over the popcorn, being careful that the cheese remains on the kernels. Bake for 3 to 4 minutes or until the cheese has melted onto the popcorn. Loosen any stuck cheese from the bottom of the pan with a broad spatula. Cool the popcorn in the pan on a wire rack. Serve immediately. Popcorn will keep for 2 to 3 days in an airtight container.

Calories 58

Calories from Fat 19

Total Fat 2 g

Saturated Fat 1 g

Cholesterol 6 mg

Sodium 69 mg

Total Carbohydrate
6 g

Dietary Fiber 1 g

Sugars 0 g

Protein 4 g

Mustard Pretzels

Preparation Time:
8 minutes

Serves 6

Serving Size:
1 cup

These tangy pretzels make a great snack. If you like a spicier pretzel, add a bit more mustard.

Nonstick cooking spray

6 cups small pretzels (about 3/16 inch in diameter)

3 Tbsp prepared mustard

1 Tbsp mild or strong honey

1/2 Tbsp cider vinegar

1/4 tsp dry mustard

1. Preheat the oven to 400 degrees. Spray a large baking pan with nonstick cooking spray. Arrange the pretzels in the pan.

2. In a small bowl, stir together the prepared mustard, honey, vinegar, and dry mustard. Slowly pour the mixture over the pretzels, stirring to coat.

3. Spread out the pretzels so that they are in 1 or 2 layers. Bake for 8 to 10 minutes, stirring once, or until the pretzels begin to brown. Cool in the pan on a wire rack until they begin to crisp. The pretzels will keep at room temperature for 1 to 2 weeks.

Exchanges
1 1/2 Starch

Calories 124

Calories from Fat 11

Total Fat 1 g

Saturated Fat 0 g

Cholesterol 0 mg

Sodium 575 mg

Total Carbohydrate 26 g

Dietary Fiber 1 g

Sugars 4 g

Protein 3 g

Garlic-Parmesan Rolls

Preparation Time:
3 minutes

Serves 2

Serving Size:
1/2 roll

If you like garlic bread, try these crispy rolls. It's most convenient to make them in the toaster oven, but you can also use the conventional oven. To speed the preparation of this recipe, I use prechopped garlic, available in the produce section of the supermarket.

1 whole-wheat or mixed-grain dinner roll
(about 1 3/4 oz)
2 tsp reduced-fat tub-style margarine
(4.5 g fat/T)
1/4–1/2 tsp chopped garlic, or to taste
Pinch basil
2 tsp grated Parmesan cheese

1. If using the conventional oven, preheat to 425 degrees.

2. Cut the roll in half. Spread each half with half the margarine and half the garlic. Sprinkle on the Parmesan cheese and press it into place with the back of a spoon.

3. If using the toaster oven, place the roll halves on the rack and crisp until browned. Serve immediately.

4. If using the conventional oven, lay the rolls on a baking sheet and bake for about 5 minutes or until browned. Serve warm.

Exchanges

1 Starch

1/2 Fat

Calories 86

Calories from Fat 30

Total Fat 3 g

Saturated Fat 1 g

Cholesterol 3 mg

Sodium 203 mg

Total Carbohydrate
12 g

Dietary Fiber 2 g

Sugars 2 g

Protein 4 g

Tortilla Pinwheels

Preparation Time:
10 minutes

Serves 2

Serving Size:
2 pieces

Before making these easy pinwheels, check the tortilla nutrition labels. While some tortillas are quite high in fat, others have almost none.

1 Tbsp fat-free cream cheese
2 Tbsp shredded reduced-fat Cheddar cheese
2 Tbsp mild salsa
1 Tbsp chopped green onion tops
1/8 tsp chili powder
1 6-inch low-fat flour tortilla

1. In a small bowl, stir together the cream cheese and Cheddar cheese with a fork until the Cheddar is incorporated. Stir in the salsa, green onion, and chili powder.

2. Spread the mixture evenly on the tortilla. Roll up and cut off the ends. Cut tortilla into 4 pieces and serve.

Exchanges

1/2 Starch
1 Very Lean Meat

Calories 70

Calories from Fat 14

Total Fat 2 g

Saturated Fat 1 g

Cholesterol 6 mg

Sodium 258 mg

Total Carbohydrate 10 g

Dietary Fiber 1 g

Sugars 1 g

Protein 5 g

Serves 2

Serving Size:
  1/2 apple and
  1/2 oz cheese

Apples and Cheese

The taste and texture of apples and cheese complement each other perfectly in this easy recipe. For an interesting variation, you can substitute a pear for the apple or blue cheese for the feta.

1 large Granny Smith apple
1 oz reduced-fat feta cheese

1. Core and slice the apple. Cut the feta into thin slices.

2. Lay the apple slices on two plates. Lay the cheese over the apple.

Exchanges

1 Fruit

1/2 Fat

Calories 84

Calories from Fat 18

Total Fat 2 g

Saturated Fat 1.3 g

Cholesterol 4 mg

Sodium 197 mg

Total Carbohydrate
  15 g

Dietary Fiber 3 g

Sugars 11 g

Protein 3 g

Asian Triangles

Preparation Time:
8 minutes

Serves 6

Serving Size:
4 pieces

These tangy triangles are fun to make and fun to eat.

Nonstick cooking spray
1 Tbsp smooth peanut butter
1/2 Tbsp lite soy sauce
1 tsp water
1/2 tsp Asian sesame oil
4 tsp rice or white vinegar
1/4 tsp ginger
2–3 drops hot pepper sauce
12 wonton wrappers, cut in half to form
      triangles

1. Preheat the oven to 400 degrees. Spray a large baking sheet with nonstick cooking spray. Set aside.

2. In a small microwave-safe bowl, combine the peanut butter, soy sauce, water, oil, vinegar, ginger, and hot pepper sauce. Microwave for 20 to 30 seconds to warm the mixture, so that peanut butter will easily combine with the other ingredients. With a small wire whisk, whisk until well combined.

3. Arrange the wonton wrappers on the baking sheet in a single layer. With your finger, brush the mixture over the top of the wonton triangles.

4. Bake for 3 to 5 minutes, or until the triangles have crisped. Cool in the pan on a wire rack, or serve warm. Triangles will keep for up to a week in an airtight container.

Exchanges
1/2 Starch
1/2 Fat

Calories 54
Calories from Fat 17
Total Fat 2 g
Saturated Fat 0 g
Cholesterol 2 mg
Sodium 131 mg
Total Carbohydrate 8 g
Dietary Fiber 1 g
Sugars 1 g
Protein 2 g

Serves 10

Serving Size:
  5 pieces

Parmesan Triangles

Try these crispy Parmesan snacks the next time your friends drop in.

Nonstick cooking spray

1 Tbsp olive oil

1 Tbsp water

1 garlic clove, minced

1 tsp Italian seasoning

25 wonton wrappers, cut in half to form triangles

2 Tbsp grated Parmesan cheese

Exchanges

1/2 Starch

1/2 Fat

Calories 61

Calories from Fat 18

Total Fat 2 g

Saturated Fat 1 g

Cholesterol 4 mg

Sodium 111 mg

Total Carbohydrate 9 g

Dietary Fiber 1 g

Sugars 0 g

Protein 2 g

1. Preheat the oven to 400 degrees. Spray a large baking sheet with nonstick cooking spray. Set aside.

2. In a small bowl, stir together the oil, water, garlic, and Italian seasoning.

3. Set the wonton wrappers on the baking sheet in a single layer.

4. With your finger, spread the oil mixture over the wonton triangles. (If the mixture begins to separate, stir again.) Sprinkle with the cheese.

5. Bake for 3 to 4 minutes until the triangles have crisped. Cool in the pan on a wire rack, or serve warm. Triangles will keep for up to a week in an airtight container.

The Bake Shop

The savory dishes in this chapter are served hot from the oven. Included is a cornbread that can be served as a snack any time, even for breakfast. I've also developed an easy dough you can use for homemade pizza or calzone, which are Italian baked turnovers. It's fun to make your own dough, but if you like, you can save time by purchasing an unbaked pizza crust.

Serves 9

Serving Size:
1 oz

Pizza or Calzone Crust

Here's an easy dough that can be used for either pizza or calzone. You can make it in a food processor or knead it by hand. Water temperature is important for good results. If the water is too hot, it will kill the yeast. If it's too cold, the yeast won't make the dough rise. Test the water-oil mixture with a candy thermometer before adding it to the flour-yeast mixture.

1 3/4 cups all-purpose white flour
1 package quick-rising yeast
3/4 tsp salt
1/2 tsp sugar
2/3 cup water (125–130°F)
1 Tbsp olive oil
Nonstick cooking spray

Exchanges

1 Starch

1/2 Fat

Calories 105

Calories from Fat 16

Total Fat 2 g

Saturated Fat 0.2 g

Cholesterol 0 mg

Sodium 195 mg

Total Carbohydrate 19 g

Dietary Fiber 1 g

Sugars 1 g

Protein 3 g

1. In a food processor container fitted with a steel blade, combine the flour, yeast, salt, and sugar. Pulse to mix. Combine hot water and olive oil and test temperature. With food processor on, gradually add the water-oil mixture through the feed tube. Process until the dough forms a ball, about 5 to 10 seconds. Then process for 1 minute longer to knead. Remove the dough from processor. If it seems sticky, work in 2 or 3 tsp of flour.

2. To mix by hand, combine the flour, yeast, salt, and sugar in a medium bowl. Combine the hot water and the oil and test temperature. With a large spoon, stir in the water-oil mixture and mix in. Knead by hand until a smooth dough is formed, about 3 to 5 minutes. If the dough

seems sticky, work in 2 or 3 additional tsp of flour.

3. Turn dough out onto a lightly floured board. Spray plastic wrap with nonstick cooking spray, cover dough, and let rise 15 minutes.

4. Preheat the oven to 425 degrees. Spray a large baking sheet or pizza pan with nonstick cooking spray. Lightly sprinkle with cornmeal, if desired. Transfer the dough to the pan. Stretch and shape the dough by hand and/or with a rolling pin into a 12- or 13-inch circle or an 11- by 14-inch rectangle. Add additional ingredients for pizza or calzone from recipes on pages 60, 62, 64, and 66. Bake for 15 to 17 minutes on center oven rack or until crust is lightly browned.

Spinach, Red Onion, and Cheese Pizza

If you like white pizza (with no tomato sauce), try this cheese and spinach version. It can be made with the dough on page 58 or on a store-bought pizza crust.

Nonstick cooking spray

1 homemade or store-bought pizza crust (see recipe, p. 58)

1 1/2 cups loose-leaf, dry-packed frozen spinach

1/4 cup chopped red onion

1/2 cup fat-free ricotta cheese

1 1/4 tsp Italian seasoning

1 garlic clove, minced

2–3 drops hot pepper sauce

1/3 cup crumbled feta cheese

2 Tbsp grated Parmesan cheese

Exchanges

1 Starch

1 Vegetable

1/2 Fat

Calories 133

Calories from Fat 29

Total Fat 3 g

Saturated Fat 1 g

Cholesterol 10 mg

Sodium 308 mg

Total Carbohydrate 20 g

Dietary Fiber 2 g

Sugars 2 g

Protein 7 g

1. Preheat the oven to 425 degrees. Spray a large baking sheet or pizza pan with nonstick cooking spray. Lightly sprinkle with cornmeal, if desired. Set aside.

2. If making the crust, transfer the dough to the pan. Stretch and shape the dough by hand or with a rolling pin into a 12- or 13-inch circle or 11- by 14-inch rectangle. If using store-bought crust, place it on the pan.

3. Place the spinach and red onion in a small microwave-safe bowl, cover with wax paper, and microwave on defrost power for 2 to 3 minutes, or until the spinach is thawed and the onion is softened.

4. Place the ricotta in a small bowl and stir in the spinach mixture, Italian seasoning, garlic, and hot pepper sauce. Spread the ricotta mixture onto the pizza dough. Sprinkle with the feta and Parmesan cheeses.

5. For homemade crust, bake for 15 to 17 minutes on center oven rack or until crust is lightly browned. For store-bought crust, bake according to package directions. Cut into 9 rectangles or wedges and serve.

Preparation Time:
20 minutes

Serves 8

Serving Size:
1 piece

Artichoke, Shrimp, and Roasted Red Pepper Pizza

Make this tasty pizza with the homemade crust on page 58, or use a store-bought pizza crust.

Nonstick cooking spray

1 homemade or store-bought pizza crust (see recipe, p. 58)

1 cup water-packed artichoke heart quarters, well drained

1 cup pizza sauce

1 1/2 cups cooked shrimp

1/4 cup roasted red pepper, chopped

2 Tbsp grated Parmesan cheese

Exchanges

1 Starch

1 Vegetable

1 Lean Meat

Calories 164

Calories from Fat 29

Total Fat 3 g

Saturated Fat 1 g

Cholesterol 49 mg

Sodium 559 mg

Total Carbohydrate 24 g

Dietary Fiber 2 g

Sugars 3 g

Protein 10 g

1. Preheat the oven to 425 degrees. Spray a large baking sheet or pizza pan with nonstick cooking spray. Lightly sprinkle with cornmeal, if desired.

2. If making the crust, transfer the dough to the pan. Stretch and shape the dough by hand or with a rolling pin into a 12- or 13-inch circle or 11- by 14-inch rectangle. If using store-bought crust, place it on the pan.

3. Remove and discard any coarse outer leaves from the artichoke hearts. Coarsely chop the hearts.

4. Spread the pizza sauce over the crust. Sprinkle the artichoke hearts evenly over the crust. Sprinkle on the shrimp and then the chopped pepper. Top with cheese.

5. Bake homemade crust for 12 to 15 minutes. If using purchased crust, bake according to package directions, or until pizza begins to brown at edges. Cut into 8 rectangles or wedges and serve.

Pizza Puffs

Here are puffy individual pizza snacks in minutes!

Nonstick cooking spray

1 1/2 Tbsp low-sodium or regular tomato sauce

Scant 1/2 tsp Italian seasoning

1 4 1/2-oz package reduced-fat refrigerator buttermilk biscuits

1/2 Tbsp grated Parmesan cheese

1. Preheat the oven to 450 degrees. Spray a small baking sheet with nonstick cooking spray. Set aside.

2. In a custard cup, mix together the tomato sauce and Italian seasoning. Set aside.

3. Open the biscuit carton and separate the biscuits. Place them on the baking sheet.

4. With a small spoon, spread the tomato sauce and seasoning mixture on the biscuits, dividing the mixture evenly. Bake in the center of the oven for 8 to 10 minutes or until golden. Serve hot.

5. Leftovers will keep for 1 to 2 days in the refrigerator, tightly wrapped.

Preparation Time: 6 minutes

Serves 6

Serving Size: 1 piece

Exchanges

1/2 Starch

Calories 54

Calories from Fat 8

Total Fat 1 g

Saturated Fat 0 g

Cholesterol 1 mg

Sodium 191 mg

Total Carbohydrate 10 g

Dietary Fiber 0 g

Sugars 1 g

Protein 2 g

Barbecued Chicken Pizza

Barbecued chicken makes a differently delicious pizza topping. Use the homemade crust on page 58 or a purchased crust. You can use leftover roast chicken or quickly cook a chicken breast in the microwave.

1 8-oz can reduced-sodium tomato sauce or regular tomato sauce

1/4 cup finely chopped onion

1 Tbsp Splenda

1/4 tsp cider vinegar

1/2 tsp dry mustard

1/4 tsp dried thyme leaves

Pinch of ground cloves

1/8 tsp black pepper

2–3 drops hot pepper sauce (optional)

3/4 cup cooked chicken breast meat, cut into very small pieces

1 large homemade or purchased pizza crust (see p. 58)

3/4 cup shredded nonfat Cheddar cheese

1. Preheat the oven to 400 degrees. In a 2-cup measure or similar microwave-safe container, combine the tomato sauce, onion, Splenda, vinegar, mustard, thyme, cloves, pepper, and hot pepper sauce, if desired. Cover with wax paper and microwave on high power for 1 1/2 to 2 minutes, until the sauce is bubbly. Stir in the chicken.

Exchanges

1 1/2 Starch

1 Very Lean Meat

1/2 Fat

Calories 167

Calories from Fat 23

Total Fat 3 g

Saturated Fat 0.4 g

Cholesterol 12 mg

Sodium 342 mg

Total Carbohydrate 25 g

Dietary Fiber 1 g

Sugars 3 g

Protein 11 g

2. Spread the sauce mixture on a large pizza crust. Sprinkle with cheese. If using homemade crust, bake for 8 to 10 minutes. If using purchased crust, bake according to package directions, or until the crust begins to brown at the edges.

Mini Spinach and Cheese Calzone

Calzone are Italian baked turnovers. I've used an easy dough (see recipe, p. 58) and a creamy spinach and cheese filling in these.

1 unbaked homemade or store-bought pizza crust (see recipe, p. 58)

Nonstick cooking spray

Cornmeal (optional)

1 1/2 cups loose-leaf, dry-pack frozen spinach

1 cup shredded reduced-fat mozzarella cheese

3/4 cup fat-free ricotta cheese

3 Tbsp grated Parmesan cheese

1 1/4 tsp Italian seasoning

1 garlic clove, minced

Pinch nutmeg

2–3 drops hot pepper sauce

1 Tbsp low-fat (1%) milk (optional)

Exchanges

1 1/2 Starch

1 Lean Meat

Calories 170

Calories from Fat 39

Total Fat 4 g

Saturated Fat 1.7 g

Cholesterol 15 mg

Sodium 346 mg

Total Carbohydrate 22 g

Dietary Fiber 2 g

Sugars 2 g

Protein 11 g

1. Prepare the basic dough according to the directions in the dough recipe (p. 58). Preheat the oven to 375 degrees. Spray a large baking sheet with nonstick cooking spray. Lightly sprinkle with cornmeal, if desired. Set aside.

2. Place the spinach in a small microwave-safe bowl. Cover with wax paper and microwave on low power for 2 to 3 minutes, or until the spinach is thawed.

3. In a large bowl, stir together the mozzarella, ricotta, Parmesan, Italian seasoning, garlic, nutmeg, and hot pepper sauce. Stir in the spinach.

4. Divide the dough into 9 equal portions. On a lightly floured board, roll each portion of the dough into a 5-inch circle, adding additional flour to the board if needed. (Hint: If the dough is difficult to roll to this diameter, roll each circle to 4 inches. Allow to rest before rolling out to the full 5 inches.) While working, stack circles on a plate, covering with plastic wrap.

5. For each calzone, spoon about 2 generous tablespoons of the filling mixture onto half of one dough circle, leaving 1/2 inch at the edge. Moisten the edges of the dough with water. Fold the dough in half over the filling. Seal by pressing with fork tines. Transfer the calzone to the prepared baking sheet. Prick the top to allow steam to escape. For a richer appearance, brush the tops of the calzone lightly with milk before baking.

6. Bake for 20 to 22 minutes on the center oven rack or until crust is lightly browned. Allow the calzone to cool 3 or 4 minutes before serving. Wrap and refrigerate leftovers for up to 3 days or freeze. Reheat in the microwave.

Serves 10

Serving Size:
1 piece

Ham and Cheese Puffs

These puffy little ham and cheese biscuits make a great snack or appetizer.

Nonstick cooking spray

1 7 1/2-oz package reduced-fat refrigerator buttermilk biscuits or rolls

3 Tbsp seasoned tomato sauce

2 Tbsp chopped reduced-fat ham or Canadian bacon

2 Tbsp reduced-fat shredded Cheddar cheese

1. Preheat the oven to 450 degrees. Spray a small baking sheet with nonstick cooking spray. Set aside.

2. Open the biscuit carton and separate the biscuits. Place them on the baking sheet.

3. With a small spoon, spread the tomato sauce on the biscuits, dividing the mixture evenly. Top with the ham and cheese, dividing evenly.

4. Bake in the center of the oven for 8 to 10 minutes or until golden. Serve hot. Leftovers will keep for 1 to 2 days in the refrigerator, tightly wrapped.

Exchanges

1/2 Starch

Calories 59

Calories from Fat 10

Total Fat 1 g

Saturated Fat 0 g

Cholesterol 2 mg

Sodium 231 mg

Total Carbohydrate 10 g

Dietary Fiber 0 g

Sugars 1 g

Protein 2 g

Tex-Mex Cornbread

Preparation Time:
18 minutes

Serves 9

Serving Size:
1 square

This spicy cornbread tastes best made with medium salsa.
If you use mild, add 2 or 3 drops of hot pepper sauce.

Nonstick cooking spray
1 cup yellow cornmeal
3/4 cup all-purpose or unbleached white flour
2 Tbsp Splenda
2 tsp baking powder
1/8 tsp salt
2 Tbsp reduced-fat margarine or butter
1/2 cup fat-free half-and-half
1/4 cup water
1/4 cup liquid egg substitute
1/3 cup medium chunky salsa

1. Preheat oven to 400 degrees. Coat an 8-inch square baking pan with nonstick cooking spray.

2. In a medium bowl combine the cornmeal, flour, Splenda, baking powder, and salt.

3. Cut in the margarine with a pastry cutter or two forks until well combined. Add the half-and-half, water, egg substitute, and salsa and stir in with a few swift strokes.

4. Transfer batter to the prepared pan and spread it out to the edges of the pan using the back of a large spoon. Bake for 17 to 21 minutes or until the cornbread is lightly browned and a toothpick inserted in the center comes out clean.

5. Serve warm. Store leftover cornbread tightly wrapped at room temperature.

Exchanges
1 1/2 Starch

Calories 119
Calories from Fat 14
Total Fat 2 g
Saturated Fat 0.2 g
Cholesterol 1 mg
Sodium 218 mg
Total Carbohydrate 22 g
Dietary Fiber 2 g
Sugars 2 g
Protein 4 g

Onion and Garlic Focaccia

This Italian peasant bread is easy and fun to make at home, but you do have to wait for the dough to rise. Water temperature is important for good results. If the water is too hot, it will kill the yeast. If it's too cold, the yeast won't make the dough rise. If you have a heavy-duty mixer equipped with a bread hook, use it to knead the dough; otherwise, knead by hand.

2 3/4–3 cups all-purpose white flour, divided
1 cup finely chopped onion
2 garlic cloves, minced
2 Tbsp olive oil
2 tsp Italian seasoning, divided
1 tsp sugar
3/4–1 tsp salt
1 packet quick-acting dry yeast
1 scant cup water (125–130°F)
3–4 drops hot pepper sauce
Nonstick cooking spray
1 Tbsp olive oil
1 cup chopped onion
1 garlic clove, minced

Calories 131

Calories from Fat 27

Total Fat 3 g

Saturated Fat 1 g

Cholesterol 0 mg

Sodium 118 mg

Total Carbohydrate
23 g

Dietary Fiber 1 g

Sugars 2 g

Protein 3 g

1. In a large mixing bowl, combine 1 1/2 cups of the flour, onion, garlic, oil, 1 tsp Italian seasoning, sugar, salt, and yeast. Add the warm water and hot pepper sauce. Beat with an electric mixer on low speed for 1 minute, scraping bowl frequently.

2. Increase the speed to medium and beat 1 minute, scraping bowl frequently. Stir in enough of

the remaining flour, 1/2 cup at a time, to make dough easy to handle. Form into a ball.

3. Use mixer bread hook to knead dough for 3 to 5 minutes until very cohesive, or turn out onto a lightly floured board and knead with lightly oiled hands for 5 to 8 minutes until very cohesive.

4. Transfer the dough to a nonstick 9 1/2- by 13-inch pan. Press and spread dough to cover bottom surface of pan, making thickness even. Cover with nonstick spray-coated plastic wrap.

5. Allow to rise in a warm place for 40 to 45 minutes, until dough has grown about 1/2 inch higher. Poke random indentations in the dough with your finger to create an uneven surface.

6. Preheat the oven to 400 degrees. Bake bread for 15 minutes. Meanwhile, in a small skillet, combine oil, onion, garlic, and 1 tsp Italian seasoning. Cook over medium heat, stirring frequently, until the onion is tender. Set aside.

7. Remove the bread from the oven and spread the onion mixture evenly over the top. Return the bread to the oven and bake an additional 15 to 20 minutes until lightly browned on top.

8. Remove the bread from the pan. Cool on a wire rack. Cut into 15 rectangles. When cooled, wrap tightly in plastic wrap. The bread will keep for 1 to 2 days at room temperature. Freeze for longer storage.

Baked Egg Rolls

Serves 12

Serving Size:
1 egg roll

It's fun to experiment at home with foods you've previously only eaten in restaurants. If you love egg rolls, here's a baked version that's far lower in calories than the deep-fried variety. About a cup of freshly chopped mushrooms can be substituted for part of the bean sprouts or cabbage.

Nonstick cooking spray

1 Tbsp lite soy sauce

1 tsp cornstarch

1/2 tsp rice or white vinegar

1/4 tsp packed brown sugar

2 tsp Asian sesame oil

1/2 cup thinly sliced green onion tops

2 cups fresh bean sprouts

2 cups finely chopped Chinese cabbage

1 cup small cooked shrimp, chopped

12 egg roll wrappers

Exchanges

1 Starch

1 Vegetable

Calories 117

Calories from Fat 13

Total Fat 1 g

Saturated Fat 0 g

Cholesterol 24 mg

Sodium 265 mg

Total Carbohydrate
21 g

Dietary Fiber 2 g

Sugars 1 g

Protein 6 g

1. Preheat the oven to 400 degrees. Spray a large baking sheet with nonstick cooking spray and set aside. In a small bowl, mix together the soy sauce, cornstarch, and vinegar until smooth. Stir in the sugar. Set aside.

2. In a large nonstick skillet, combine the oil, onion, bean sprouts, and cabbage. Cook over medium-high heat, stirring frequently, for about 3 minutes, or until the vegetables are softened. Stir in the reserved cornstarch mixture and the shrimp and cook for 1 or 2 minutes longer or until the sauce has thickened. Remove to a strainer and drain off excess liquid.

3. To fill each egg roll, lay a wrapper on a flat surface with one corner facing you. Lay about 3 Tbsp of filling in a line horizontally across the center of the wrapper, leaving about 1 1/2 inches at each pointed end. Fold the pointed end of the wrapper facing you over the filling. Fold in the pointed ends at the sides of the wrapper over the filling.

4. Brush the remaining pointed end of the wrapper with cold water. Fold the remaining end of the wrapper over the filling, rolling to make the traditional egg roll shape. Transfer to the baking sheet. Spray the egg rolls lightly with nonstick cooking spray.

5. Bake for 13 minutes, or until the wrappers are crisped. The egg rolls are best served hot from the oven. Egg rolls can be cooled, covered, and refrigerated for up to 24 hours before serving. Rewarm in a 350-degree oven for 9 to 11 minutes.

Herbed Crackers

Preparation Time:
20 minutes

Serves 17

Serving Size:
2 crackers

Exchanges

1/2 Starch

Calories 35

Calories from Fat 13

Total Fat 1 g

Saturated Fat 0 g

Cholesterol 0 mg

Sodium 57 mg

Total Carbohydrate
5 g

Dietary Fiber 0 g

Sugars 1 g

Protein 1 g

Yes, you really can bake your own crackers instead of getting them out of a package. These are so flavorful that they need no topping. However, if you like, you can serve them with some cheese or a spread.

Nonstick cooking spray
1/2 cup plus 1 Tbsp white flour
1/3 cup oat bran
1 tsp instant minced onions
1 garlic clove, minced
1/4 tsp baking soda
1/4 tsp dried thyme leaves
1/2 tsp basil
1/4 tsp salt
Pinch white pepper
1 1/2 Tbsp olive oil
1/4 cup low-fat buttermilk

1. Preheat the oven to 350 degrees. Spray a large baking sheet that is rimless on at least 2 sides with nonstick cooking spray. Or use the back of a rimmed baking sheet.

2. In a medium bowl, combine the flour, oat bran, onions, garlic, baking soda, thyme, basil, salt, and pepper.

3. Stir to mix well. Add the oil and buttermilk, and stir with a large spoon until thoroughly combined. If necessary, work in the last of the flour mixture with your fingertips. Gather the dough into a ball.

4. Place the dough ball on the prepared baking sheet. Cover with wax paper and roll the dough into a 10- by 14-inch rectangle. Try to keep the thickness of the dough as even as possible, as thick crackers will not be as crisp. Cut and patch the dough if necessary to make the sides of the rectangle straight. Gently peel off and discard the wax paper immediately after rolling out the dough.

5. Prick the dough all over with the tines of a fork. Then use a sharp knife, pizza cutter, or pastry wheel to cut the rolled-out dough into squares about 1 1/2 by 2 inches on a side, leaving the dough in place on the baking sheet.

6. Bake in the center of the oven for 12 to 15 minutes, or until the crackers on the edges of the sheet are lightly browned and crisp. Remove the baking sheet from the oven and separate the browned crackers from the rest of the sheet with a metal spatula.

7. Transfer the browned crackers to a wire rack to cool and return the baking sheet to the oven. Continue baking, checking the crackers about every 1 1/2 to 2 minutes and removing them from the sheet when they are done.

8. Continue until all of the crackers are lightly browned. When the crackers are slightly cooled, separate any that are still stuck together. Cool completely on a metal rack. Crackers will keep for up to a week in an airtight container.

Crowd Pleasers

There are times when you don't want to fuss with a sit-down meal, but you do want to serve snacks that guests can enjoy. If the guys are coming over for the Super Bowl, give them Bean and Pasta Soup with Sausage, Chili Con Queso, or Black and Red Bean Tortilla Bake.

Or, for the ladies' bridge club, set out Salmon Mousse or Stuffed Artichoke Hearts. For an afternoon open house, try Cocktail Meatballs, Italian Chicken Nuggets, or Stuffed Mushrooms. Almost all of the recipes in the chapter are easily doubled if you want to feed an even larger crowd.

Notice that I've come up with a sneaky way to make better-for-you meatballs. Instead of using all ground beef, I've mixed in some ground turkey breast meat. When combined this way, the turkey takes on the flavor of the beef, and even ground turkey haters like my husband can't detect it.

The secret is in using a mixture of slightly less than half ground turkey breast. And be sure to use turkey breast, since it's far lower in fat than "lean" ground turkey, which contains high-fat dark meat and skin.

When I buy ground turkey, I use some at once and divide the rest into 4- to 6-ounce portions that I freeze for later use.

Bean and Pasta Soup with Sausage

Here's an easy but delicious bean soup that cooks quickly and can be packed in a thermos and taken to a football game or fall tailgate picnic. You can also serve it for a quick lunch or dinner entrée.

1 medium onion, chopped

1 large celery stalk, minced

1 garlic clove, minced

2 tsp olive oil

3 cups fat-free, low-sodium or regular chicken broth, divided

1 15-oz can cannellini beans, rinsed and well drained

1 8-oz can low-sodium or regular tomato sauce

1 tsp Italian seasoning

2–3 drops hot pepper sauce (optional)

3 oz reduced-fat beef sausage

1 oz angel hair pasta broken into 2-inch pieces (about 1/2 cup)

Salt to taste (optional)

1. In a small Dutch oven or similar pot, combine the onion, celery, garlic, oil, and 1/4 cup broth. Cook over medium heat, stirring frequently, for 6 to 7 minutes or until the onion is tender.

2. Add remaining broth, beans, tomato sauce, Italian seasoning, and hot pepper sauce (if desired). Bring to a boil over high heat. Reduce heat and simmer, uncovered, stirring occasionally, for 15 minutes.

3. Bring soup to a boil. Stir in sausage and pasta. Reduce heat and cook at a low boil for 4 or 5 minutes until the pasta is tender. Add salt to taste, if desired.

Preparation Time: 20 minutes

Serves 6

Serving Size: 3/4 cup

Exchanges

1 Starch

1 Vegetable

1 Very Lean Meat

Calories 147

Calories from Fat 21

Total Fat 2 g

Saturated Fat 0 g

Cholesterol 6 mg

Sodium 573 mg

Total Carbohydrate 23 g

Dietary Fiber 4 g

Sugars 5 g

Protein 9 g

Bean and Corn Con Carne Soup

Here's another quick but hearty soup that's perfect for the football crowd. While there's only a little meat in the soup, it lends both flavor and texture.

1/2 lb reduced-fat ground beef

1 large onion, finely chopped

3 3/4 cups beef broth (2 14 1/2-oz cans)

1 14 1/2-oz can low-sodium or regular stewed tomatoes

2 15 1/2-oz cans low-sodium or regular kidney beans, rinsed and well drained

1 1/2 cups loose-pack frozen corn kernels

2 tsp chili powder, or to taste

1 tsp cumin

1/4 tsp black pepper

1/2 tsp salt or to taste (optional)

Exchanges

1 1/2 Starch

1 Vegetable

1 Very Lean Meat

Calories 167

Calories from Fat 16

Total Fat 2 g

Saturated Fat 0 g

Cholesterol 14 mg

Sodium 373 mg

Total Carbohydrate 26 g

Dietary Fiber 6 g

Sugars 5 g

Protein 13 g

1. In a large, heavy pot, combine the ground beef and onion. Cook over medium heat, stirring frequently and breaking up the meat with a large spoon, for 5 to 6 minutes or until browned. If the meat sticks to the pot, add a small amount of the broth.

2. Add the broth, tomatoes, beans, corn, chili powder, cumin, pepper, and salt (if desired). Stir to mix well.

3. Bring the soup to a boil. Cover the pot, lower the heat, and simmer for 20 to 25 minutes, stirring occasionally. With a large, shallow spoon, skim off and discard any fat from the top of the soup.

4. Serve at once, or refrigerate and rewarm. This soup keeps for 4 to 5 days in the refrigerator.

West African Sweet Potato–Peanut Soup

Expand your horizons with this simple but very tasty soup. The recipe calls for nonfat half-and-half, which adds a very creamy taste to the soup.

2 celery stalks, diced

1/4 cup chopped onion

1 garlic clove, minced

4 cups fat-free, reduced-sodium chicken broth, divided

2 Tbsp natural (nonhydrogenated, no-sugar) peanut butter

1 1/4 tsp ground cumin

1/8 tsp ground celery seed

1/8 tsp ground white pepper, or to taste

1 large (15–16 oz) sweet potato, cooked

1/4 cup nonfat half-and-half

1. In a large saucepan, combine the celery, onion, and garlic with 1 cup of the broth. Bring to a boil. Reduce the heat and simmer, covered, for 8 to 10 minutes, until softened.

2. Whisk the peanut butter into the broth and vegetable mixture, until well combined. Stir in 1 cup of additional broth. Stir in the cumin, celery seed, and pepper.

3. Scoop out the sweet potato meat and stir it into the soup. Use the whisk or a potato masher to partially break up the sweet potato. Add the remaining broth. Bring to a boil, reduce the heat, and simmer, covered, for 5 to 7 minutes, until the flavors are well blended. Stir in the half-and-half and cook an additional minute. Serve hot.

Preparation Time: 20 minutes

Serves 4

Serving Size: 1 cup

Exchanges

2 Carbohydrate

1/2 Fat

Calories 170

Calories from Fat 42

Total Fat 5 g

Saturated Fat 0.9 g

Cholesterol 1 mg

Sodium 579 mg

Total Carbohydrate 26 g

Dietary Fiber 3 g

Sugars 7 g

Protein 7 g

Italian Chicken Nuggets

Preparation Time:
18 minutes

Serves 14

Serving Size:
2 nuggets

These bite-sized, crispy-tender chicken pieces are especially good with a dipping sauce, such as low-fat Italian dressing, barbecue sauce, or the Tangy Mustard Sauce on page 159. To speed preparation, you can coat the chicken with the sour cream mixture in advance and refrigerate for up to 6 hours.

Nonstick cooking spray

1/4 cup fat-free sour cream

1 tsp Italian seasoning

1/4 tsp salt, or to taste (optional)

2–3 drops hot pepper sauce

1 lb boneless, skinless chicken breast, cut into bite-sized pieces

1/2 cup Italian-style commercial bread crumbs

Exchanges

1 Lean Meat

Calories 58

Calories from Fat 8

Total Fat 1 g

Saturated Fat 0 g

Cholesterol 20 mg

Sodium 139 mg

Total Carbohydrate 4 g

Dietary Fiber 0 g

Sugars 1 g

Protein 8 g

1. Preheat the oven to 450 degrees. Coat a large baking sheet with nonstick cooking spray and set aside.

2. In a large bowl, combine the sour cream, Italian seasoning, salt (if desired), and hot pepper sauce. Stir to mix well. Stir in the chicken pieces and stir to coat well.

3. Place the bread crumbs in a medium bowl. Roll the chicken pieces a few at a time in the bread crumbs. Set pieces on baking sheet. Bake in preheated oven for 7 to 9 minutes or until the chicken is cooked through but still moist. Serve warm, with toothpicks.

4. Cover and refrigerate leftovers, which will keep for 1 to 2 days in the refrigerator.

Chili Con Queso Dip

Preparation Time:
18 minutes

Serves 32

Serving Size:
2 Tbsp and
4 chips

Here's a crowd pleaser you'll serve frequently.

5 oz lean ground beef

4 oz ground turkey breast

2 cups frozen mixed pepper and onion stir-fry

1 garlic clove, minced

1 16-oz jar mild salsa

1 8-oz can low-sodium or regular tomato sauce

2 Tbsp tomato paste

1 tsp chili powder

1 tsp cumin

1/2 tsp salt, or to taste (optional)

1 cup grated reduced-fat Cheddar cheese

4 fat-free tortilla chips per person

1. In a small Dutch oven or large pot, combine the ground beef, ground turkey, pepper and onion mixture, and garlic. Cook over medium heat until the beef is brown, breaking up any large pieces of onion, about 5 to 6 minutes.

2. Add the salsa, tomato sauce, tomato paste, chili powder, cumin, and salt (if desired). Stir to mix well. Cover and simmer for 15 minutes, stirring frequently, to allow the flavors to blend. Remove from the heat. Stir in the cheese until melted.

3. Serve warm in a chafing dish or on a hot plate. Serve with fat-free tortilla chips. Cover and refrigerate leftovers. Leftovers keep for 3 to 4 days in the refrigerator.

Exchanges

1/2 Starch

Calories 47

Calories from Fat 10

Total Fat 1 g

Saturated Fat 1 g

Cholesterol 7 mg

Sodium 97 mg

Total Carbohydrate 6 g

Dietary Fiber 1 g

Sugars 1 g

Protein 4 g

Cocktail Meatballs

Preparation Time:
45 minutes

Serves 34

Serving Size:
2 meatballs

Exchanges

1 Very Lean Meat

Calories 36

Calories from Fat 5

Total Fat 1 g

Saturated Fat 0 g

Cholesterol 12 mg

Sodium 11 mg

Total Carbohydrate
3 g

Dietary Fiber 0 g

Sugars 1 g

Protein 5 g

These wonderful meatballs taste like they're all beef, but they're a lot healthier because they contain fresh ground turkey breast. Mixed with lean ground beef, the turkey takes on a beefy flavor and is virtually undetectable. Don't substitute ordinary ground turkey, as it contains fatty dark meat and sometimes skin.

Meatballs:
Nonstick cooking spray
1 lb reduced-fat ground beef
9 oz fresh ground turkey breast
1/2 cup quick-cooking rolled oats
1 medium onion, finely chopped
1 garlic clove, minced
1 tsp dried thyme leaves
1 tsp dried marjoram leaves
1 large egg white
1/2 tsp salt (optional)
1/8 tsp black pepper

Sauce:
1 15-oz can low-sodium or regular tomato sauce
1/2 cup water
2 Tbsp packed brown sugar
1 Tbsp balsamic vinegar
1 garlic clove, minced
3/4 tsp dry mustard
2–3 drops hot pepper sauce
1/4 tsp allspice

1. Preheat the oven to 400 degrees. Spray the bottom and sides of a large baking pan with nonstick cooking spray. Set aside.

2. In a large bowl, combine the ground beef, ground turkey, oats, onion, garlic, thyme, marjoram, egg white, salt (if desired), and pepper. Mix well. Roll into 68 1-inch balls.

3. Place the balls on the baking pan. Bake for 10 to 13 minutes, or until the meatballs are browned on all sides, turning once during browning.

4. Meanwhile, in a Dutch oven or similar heavy pot, mix together the tomato sauce, water, brown sugar, vinegar, garlic, mustard, hot pepper sauce, and allspice.

5. When the meatballs are browned, transfer them to the sauce with a large slotted spoon, cover, and bring to a boil. Reduce the heat and simmer for 30 to 35 minutes, stirring occasionally and being careful not to break up the balls. Skim any fat from the surface of the liquid.

6. Serve immediately, or cover and refrigerate. Meatballs can be refrigerated for 2 to 3 days before serving or frozen for up to a month.

Hawaiian Meatballs

Preparation Time:
35 minutes

Serves 21

Serving Size:
2 meatballs

Exchanges

1/2 Fruit

1 Very Lean Meat

Calories 56

Calories from Fat 7

Total Fat 1 g

Saturated Fat 0 g

Cholesterol 18 mg

Sodium 71 mg

Total Carbohydrate
4 g

Dietary Fiber 0 g

Sugars 4 g

Protein 8 g

The surprise ingredient in these tasty meatballs is pumpkin pie spice! Like the meatballs in the previous recipe, they combine ground turkey breast with lean ground beef, although the addition of the turkey is undetectable in the finished meatballs.

Meatballs:
1 lb reduced-fat ground beef
8 oz ground turkey breast
1 small onion, finely chopped
2 garlic cloves, minced
1/4 cup quick-cooking rolled oats
1 large egg white
1 tsp pumpkin pie spice
1 tsp dried thyme leaves
1/4 tsp salt, or to taste (optional)
Pinch black pepper
Nonstick cooking spray

Sauce:
1 1/2 cups orange juice
1 8-oz can crushed pineapple
2 Tbsp lite soy sauce
1/2 Tbsp packed light brown sugar
1/2 tsp ginger
1/8 tsp salt (optional)

SNACK MUNCH NIBBLE NOSH

1. Preheat the oven to 375 degrees. In a large bowl, combine the ground beef, ground turkey, onion, garlic, oats, egg white, pumpkin pie spice, thyme, salt (if desired), and pepper. Mix well.

2. Roll the meat mixture into about 42 balls and arrange in a large nonstick spray-coated baking pan. Bake in the upper half of the oven for 12 to 15 minutes or until browned, turning once during browning.

3. Meanwhile, combine the orange juice, pineapple, soy sauce, brown sugar, ginger, and salt (if desired) in a 3-quart flame-proof casserole. Heat the ingredients to a simmer.

4. With a large slotted spoon, transfer the meatballs to the sauce mixture and simmer, uncovered, stirring occasionally. Continue simmering for about 30 to 35 minutes, until the sauce has cooked down and thickened so that it coats the meatballs.

5. Serve at once, or cover and refrigerate. Meatballs will keep in the refrigerator for 3 to 4 days.

Serves 10

Serving Size:
3 pieces

Middle Eastern–Style Chicken

Serve these spicy chicken bits in a casserole on a hot tray or in a chafing dish. For a buffet variation, you can serve the chicken and sauce over couscous.

Nonstick cooking spray

1 lb boneless, skinless chicken breast, trimmed of all fat and cut into bite-sized pieces

2 cups frozen mixed pepper and onion stir-fry

2 garlic cloves, minced

2 tsp olive oil

1 cup fat-free, low-sodium or regular chicken broth

1 14 1/2-oz can low-sodium or regular diced tomato

1/2 cup dark raisins

1 large bay leaf

1 1/2 tsp dried thyme leaves

1 tsp cumin

1/4 tsp allspice

1/8 tsp cloves

1/8 tsp black pepper

Salt to taste (optional)

Exchanges

1/2 Carbohydrate

1 Lean Meat

Calories 99

Calories from Fat 20

Total Fat 2 g

Saturated Fat 0 g

Cholesterol 27 mg

Sodium 106 mg

Total Carbohydrate 9 g

Dietary Fiber 1 g

Sugars 7 g

Protein 11 g

1. In a nonstick skillet coated with nonstick cooking spray, cook the chicken pieces over medium heat, turning frequently, until they begin to brown.

2. Add the onion and pepper mixture, garlic, oil, and 1 Tbsp of the broth to the skillet. Stir up any browned bits from the bottom of the pan. Raise the heat and bring to a boil.

3. Lower heat again and cook over medium heat, stirring frequently, for 2 or 3 minutes, or until the onion is slightly softened. Add the remaining broth, tomato, raisins, bay leaf, thyme, cumin, allspice, cloves, and black pepper.

4. Bring to a boil, reduce the heat, and simmer, uncovered, for about 20 minutes, or until the chicken is tender and the sauce has cooked down slightly. Remove the bay leaf and discard. Add salt to taste (if desired).

5. Serve at once, or transfer to a casserole, cover, and refrigerate. The chicken will keep for 2 to 3 days in the refrigerator.

Preparation Time:
15 minutes

Serves 12

Serving Size:
1 piece

Exchanges

1 1/2 Starch

1 Vegetable

1 Very Lean Meat

Calories 191

Calories from Fat 13

Total Fat 1 g

Saturated Fat 0.4 g

Cholesterol 4 mg

Sodium 487 mg

Total Carbohydrate
29 g

Dietary Fiber 6 g

Sugars 7 g

Protein 16 g

Black and Red Bean Tortilla Bake

Tex-Mex flavors predominate in this easy layered bake. It's great as part of a buffet or when you want to feed a gang of hungry snackers.

Bake:

2 cups frozen mixed pepper and onion stir-fry

1 cup mild salsa

1 15-oz can no-salt-added tomato sauce

1 1/2 tsp cumin

1 tsp chili powder

1 15-oz can black beans, rinsed and well-drained

1 16-oz can no-salt-added kidney beans, or regular kidney beans, rinsed and well-drained

12 6-inch corn tortillas

1 1/2 cups low-fat (1%) cottage cheese

2 cups shredded fat-free Cheddar cheese, divided

Garnish:

1 large tomato, chopped

1/4 cup thinly sliced green onion tops

1/2 cup fat-free or reduced-fat sour cream

1. Preheat the oven to 350 degrees. Place the pepper-onion mixture in a 2-cup measure or similar microwave-safe bowl and cover with wax paper. Microwave on the defrost setting until the vegetables are soft, about 3 to 4 minutes. Drain in a sieve and reserve.

2. In a medium-size bowl, combine the salsa, tomato sauce, cumin, and chili powder. Stir

in the black beans, kidney beans, and reserved pepper mixture.

3. Spread one half of the bean mixture evenly in the bottom of a 9 1/2- by 13-inch baking pan. Top with one half of the tortillas in an overlapping layer. With the back of a large spoon, spread the cottage cheese evenly over the tortillas.

4. Top with one half of the Cheddar cheese. Add the remaining tortillas and then the remaining bean mixture. Cover with aluminum foil and bake for 30 to 35 minutes or until heated through.

5. Remove the aluminum foil and sprinkle the bake with the remaining Cheddar cheese. Bake, uncovered, for an additional 5 to 6 minutes or until the cheese is partially melted. To serve, cut into 12 rectangles and garnish with tomatoes, green onion, and sour cream.

Greek-Style Pizza

Serves 9

Serving Size:
1/9 of pizza

Interestingly, when I traveled around Greece, I encountered lots of small restaurants that serve pizza and other Italian-style dishes. Perhaps the Greeks acquired the habit when they were occupied by the Italians during World War II. Below is a different twist on the pizza theme—a pizza that dishes up Greek-style flavor. Note that there is no tomato sauce.

Nonstick cooking spray

Cornmeal (optional)

1 large homemade or store-bought pizza crust
(see recipe, p. 58)

Topping:

1 Tbsp olive oil

Exchanges

1 1/2 Starch

1 Vegetable

1 Lean Meat

1 medium onion (6 oz), chopped

3 cups cut-leaf, loose-pack frozen spinach

1 tsp dried dill weed

1/8 tsp salt (optional)

1/8 tsp black pepper

1/2 cup crumbled fat-free feta cheese

1 cup shredded, reduced-fat mozzarella cheese

Calories 186

Calories from Fat 48

Total Fat 5 g

Saturated Fat 1.6 g

Cholesterol 11 mg

Sodium 478 mg

Total Carbohydrate
25 g

Dietary Fiber 3 g

Sugars 2 g

Protein 11 g

1. Preheat oven to 400 degrees. Spray a large baking sheet or pizza pan with nonstick cooking spray. Lightly sprinkle with cornmeal, if desired.

2. In a medium-sized nonstick skillet, heat oil over medium heat. Cook the onion, stirring frequently, until it is soft but not browned. Stir in the spinach. Cover and cook gently for 4 to 5 minutes, stirring occasionally and breaking up any large lumps of spinach if necessary.

3. Remove the skillet from the burner. Stir in the dill, salt (if desired), and pepper.

4. Spread the spinach mixture over the pizza crust. Sprinkle the cheeses evenly over the top.

5. If using homemade crust, bake for 8 to 10 minutes. If using purchased crust, bake according to package directions or until the pizza begins to brown at the edges. Cut into 9 slices.

Salmon Mousse

Serves 16

Serving Size:
2 Tbsp

This salmon mousse looks very elegant when served in a fish mold. And the flavor is wonderful. Serve it with fat-free crackers or thinly sliced French bread. If you use a fish mold with a rounded bottom, check ahead of time to see that the mold will remain upright when the mousse is poured in. If not, make a supporting nest of crumpled aluminum foil.

1 15-oz can red salmon, drained

1 envelope unflavored gelatin

1/4 cup cold water

1/3 cup boiling water

1/4 cup reduced-fat mayonnaise

1/4 cup reduced-fat Neufchâtel cheese, at room temperature, cut into 3 or 4 pieces

3 Tbsp thinly sliced green onion tops

Exchanges

1 Lean Meat

2 Tbsp lemon juice

2 3/4 tsp fresh dill leaves or 1 tsp dried dill weed

2 tsp prepared white horseradish

Calories 53

1/4 tsp salt, or to taste (optional)

Calories from Fat 28

3–4 drops hot pepper sauce

Total Fat 3 g

1/4 cup finely chopped fresh parsley

Nonstick cooking spray

Saturated Fat 1 g

Cholesterol 16 mg

1. Remove the skin and bones from the salmon. Break the salmon meat into small pieces. Set aside in a medium bowl.

Sodium 156 mg

Total Carbohydrate
1 g

Dietary Fiber 0 g

Sugars 0 g

2. In a small bowl, sprinkle the gelatin over the cold water. Let stand for 5 minutes to soften. Add the boiling water and stir to dissolve.

Protein 5 g

3. In a food processor container, combine the salmon, mayonnaise, Neufchâtel, onion, lemon juice, dill, horseradish, salt (if desired), hot pepper sauce, and gelatin mixture. Process until almost completely smooth. Stir in the parsley.

4. Pour into a nonstick spray–coated 2- to 3-cup fish mold or other mold. Cover with plastic wrap and chill until firm, at least 4 hours or overnight. If the fish mold is unstable, lay on a plate and support with crumpled aluminum foil to keep the mold upright.

5. To unmold, run a thin knife around the edge of the mold. Dip the top of the mold in a pan of hot water for just a few seconds. Wipe dry and cover the mold with a serving platter. Invert. If necessary, shake to loosen mold.

6. Garnish with parsley or watercress. Serve with nonfat crackers. The leftover salmon mousse can be covered and refrigerated for 3 to 4 days.

Serves 28

Serving Size:
2 Tbsp

Mexican Layered Spread

This full-flavored Mexican spread is a big hit at parties. Serve the spread with fat-free tortilla chips or toasted whole-wheat pita triangles.

1 16-oz can fat-free refried beans
1 cup fat-free sour cream
1 cup mild chunky salsa
1 cup shredded reduced-fat Cheddar cheese
1–3 Tbsp thinly sliced green onion tops

1. Place the beans in a 9-inch pie plate, spreading them out evenly with the back of a serving spoon. Spread the sour cream evenly over the beans.

2. Spread the salsa evenly over the sour cream. Sprinkle evenly with the cheese. Top with the sliced green onion.

3. Serve at once, or cover and refrigerate for 2 to 3 hours or up to 24 hours before serving. The spread will keep for 3 to 4 days in the refrigerator.

Exchanges

1/2 Starch

Calories 37

Calories from Fat 8

Total Fat 1 g

Saturated Fat 1 g

Cholesterol 3 mg

Sodium 138 mg

Total Carbohydrate 4 g

Dietary Fiber 1 g

Sugars 1 g

Protein 3 g

Stuffed Artichoke Hearts

Preparation Time:
15 minutes

Serves 8

Serving Size:
1 artichoke heart

Here's the kind of recipe I like: delicious, quick, easy, and elegant. The recipe is simple to double if you want to make a larger batch.

1/3 cup chopped ripe tomato

2 Tbsp chopped chives or sliced green onion tops

1 Tbsp grated Parmesan cheese

1 tsp olive oil

Dash salt, or to taste (optional)

2 drops hot pepper sauce (optional)

1 14-oz can whole artichoke hearts, well drained

1. In a small bowl, mix together the tomato, chives, Parmesan cheese, and oil. Add the hot pepper sauce and salt, if desired.

2. Remove coarse outer leaves from the artichokes. Cut a small sliver from the bottom of the hearts so that they will stand upright. Set the artichoke hearts, bottom side down, on a plate.

3. Carefully open the leaves to form a cavity. Spoon the stuffing into the cavity in the hearts, dividing evenly.

4. Serve at once or cover and refrigerate for several hours or overnight before serving.

Exchanges

1 Vegetable

Calories 22

Calories from Fat 9

Total Fat 1 g

Saturated Fat 0 g

Cholesterol 1 mg

Sodium 104 mg

Total Carbohydrate 3 g

Dietary Fiber 1 g

Sugars 1 g

Protein 1 g

Feta-Stuffed New Potatoes

If you like the taste of feta cheese, you'll love these tiny, stuffed potato snacks.

Preparation Time:
25 minutes

Serves 8

Serving Size:
2 potato halves

8 new brown- or red-skinned potatoes no larger than 1 1/2 inches in diameter, scrubbed but not peeled

1/4 cup crumbled feta cheese

1/4 cup fat-free sour cream

1 Tbsp reduced-fat mayonnaise

1 large celery stalk, finely chopped

1 Tbsp chopped chives

1. In a steamer, steam the potatoes for 17 to 19 minutes, or until just barely tender. Meanwhile, while potatoes are cooking, in a small bowl combine the feta, sour cream, mayonnaise, celery, and chives. Stir to mix well. Set aside.

2. When the potatoes are tender, cool slightly under cold running water. Cut the potatoes in half. Cut a small slice off the rounded part of each half so that the half will stand upright. With a melon baller or small spoon, hollow out the center of each potato half, leaving a 1/4-inch-thick wall. (Reserve the potato centers for another use, if desired.)

3. Fill the potatoes with the cheese mixture and serve. Or cover and refrigerate for up to 24 hours before serving. The stuffed potatoes will keep in the refrigerator for 2 to 3 days.

Exchanges

1/2 Starch

1/2 Fat

Calories 58

Calories from Fat 12

Total Fat 1 g

Saturated Fat 1 g

Cholesterol 4 mg

Sodium 76 mg

Total Carbohydrate 9 g

Dietary Fiber 1 g

Sugars 2 g

Protein 2 g

Stuffed Mushrooms

Preparation Time:
15 minutes

Serves 10

Serving Size:
1 mushroom

Always a hit, these stuffed mushrooms are a snap to prepare. If you wash them, be sure to dry them thoroughly before stuffing them.

Nonstick cooking spray

1 lb large white mushrooms (about 10–12), cleaned and well dried with paper towels

2 Tbsp chopped chives or thinly sliced green onion tops

2 Tbsp reduced-fat mayonnaise

3 Tbsp fat-free sour cream

2 Tbsp grated Parmesan cheese

5 Tbsp Italian seasoned bread crumbs

1 Tbsp balsamic vinegar

2–3 drops hot pepper sauce (optional)

1. Preheat the broiler. Spray a baking sheet with nonstick spray. Trim the mushroom stems. Pull out the stems, chop, and reserve. Lay the mushrooms, rounded side down, on the baking sheet.

2. In a small bowl, combine 1/3 cup of the mushroom stems, chives, mayonnaise, sour cream, cheese, bread crumbs, vinegar, and hot pepper sauce (if desired). Stir to mix well.

3. Stuff each mushroom with the cheese mixture. Broil 2 inches from the broiler until the stuffing begins to brown, about 2 to 4 minutes. Serve warm.

Exchanges

1 Vegetable

1/2 Fat

Calories 41

Calories from Fat 14

Total Fat 2 g

Saturated Fat 1 g

Cholesterol 3 mg

Sodium 159 mg

Total Carbohydrate 5 g

Dietary Fiber 0 g

Sugars 1 g

Protein 2 g

Serves 18

Serving Size:
2 Tbsp

Shrimp Remoulade

These shrimp in spicy sauce make an elegant appetizer. Serve them on fat-free crackers or thin slices of French bread.

1/2 cup chili sauce

1/4 cup fat-free sour cream

2 Tbsp reduced-fat mayonnaise

1 garlic clove, minced

1 tsp prepared white horseradish

1 lb medium cooked shrimp, shelled and deveined

1. In a medium bowl, whisk together the chili sauce, sour cream, mayonnaise, garlic, and horseradish.

2. Stir in the shrimp. Serve immediately, or cover and refrigerate for several hours before serving.

Exchanges

1 Very Lean Meat

Calories 41

Calories from Fat 7

Total Fat 1 g

Saturated Fat 0 g

Cholesterol 50 mg

Sodium 162 mg

Total Carbohydrate
2 g

Dietary Fiber 0 g

Sugars 1 g

Protein 6 g

Vegetable Delights

This chapter answers the question, "Can vegetables be snacks?" Of course! Not only are they tasty, but they're the perfect health-conscious alternative to less nutritious treats. Try the Roasted Asparagus, Pan-Grilled Italian Vegetables, or Luscious Limas, and I'm sure you'll agree. All of these recipes are low in fat and calories and high in fiber. And the Portobello Mushroom Slices are heavenly—good enough to serve at the fanciest party.

Preparation Time:
2 minutes

Serves 1

Serving Size:
3 oz

Portobello Mushroom Slices

Portobello mushrooms—pan grilled and tossed with a little balsamic vinegar and Parmesan cheese. Mmm, mmm, good!

Nonstick cooking spray

3 oz portobello mushroom slices (about 8 large slices)

1 tsp olive oil

Pinch salt (optional)

1/8 tsp black pepper

1 tsp balsamic vinegar

1 tsp grated Parmesan cheese

1. Spray a medium nonstick skillet with nonstick cooking spray. Add the mushrooms to the skillet and brush with the oil, using a brush or your finger. Sprinkle with salt, if desired, and pepper.

2. Cook over medium to medium-high heat for 6 to 7 minutes or until the mushrooms have exuded their juices, softened, and begun to brown.

3. Remove the pan from the heat. Stir in the vinegar and cheese and toss to coat the mushrooms. Serve at once.

Exchanges

1 Vegetable

1 Fat

Calories 74

Calories from Fat 49

Total Fat 5 g

Saturated Fat 0.9 g

Cholesterol 2 mg

Sodium 19 mg

Total Carbohydrate 5 g

Dietary Fiber 1 g

Sugars 2 g

Protein 3 g

Florentine Potato Pancakes

Preparation Time:
6 minutes

Serves 4

Serving Size:
1 pancake

These potato pancakes get a quick start because the potatoes are first microwaved. You could omit the olive oil from the recipe if you wanted to. However, the pancakes will brown better with the oil.

2 medium red-skinned potatoes, scrubbed
1/4 cup fat-free milk
1/4 cup loose-leaf, dry-packed frozen spinach
1/2 tsp instant minced onion
Dash garlic powder
1/4 tsp salt, or to taste (optional)
1/8 tsp black pepper, or to taste
1 tsp olive oil
1/2 Tbsp grated Parmesan cheese

1. Pierce the potatoes with a fork and microwave for 7 to 8 minutes on high power, turning once, until cooked through.

2. Cut the potatoes into large chunks and transfer them to a medium bowl. Mash with a potato masher or fork. Stir in the milk, spinach, onion, garlic, salt (if desired), and pepper. Stir to mix well. Shape mixture into 4 pancakes.

3. Coat a large nonstick skillet with the oil. Cook the pancakes over medium-high heat, until browned on one side, about 2 to 3 minutes. Turn with a spatula and brown the other side.

4. Transfer the pancakes to plates and sprinkle with the Parmesan cheese, dividing it evenly. Serve hot. The pancakes will keep for 2 to 3 days in the refrigerator.

Exchanges
1 Starch

Calories 85
Calories from Fat 13
Total Fat 1 g
Saturated Fat 0 g
Cholesterol 1 mg
Sodium 40 mg
Total Carbohydrate 15 g
Dietary Fiber 2 g
Sugars 2 g
Protein 3 g

Preparation Time:
5 minutes

Serves 2

Serving Size:
5 spears and
1 oz bread

Roasted Asparagus

Once you try roasted asparagus, you'll never want to cook it any other way. This easy but elegant recipe makes a delicious snack as well as a great buffet table entrée. And it's a wonderful way to include vegetables in your meal plan.

10 medium asparagus spears, well washed and coarse ends snapped off

1 tsp olive oil

1/8 tsp salt (optional)

1/2 Tbsp grated Parmesan cheese

2 thin slices toasted Italian bread

1. Preheat the oven to 400 degrees. Dry the asparagus on paper towels. Place the spears in a shallow roasting pan. Drizzle the spears with oil and turn to coat. Sprinkle on salt (if desired).

2. Roast for 10 minutes or until the spears are tender. Remove to a plate and sprinkle with Parmesan cheese. Serve on toasted Italian bread slices.

Exchanges

1 Starch

1 Vegetable

1/2 Fat

Calories 120

Calories from Fat 37

Total Fat 4 g

Saturated Fat 1 g

Cholesterol 2 mg

Sodium 192 mg

Total Carbohydrate 17 g

Dietary Fiber 2 g

Sugars 2 g

Protein 5 g

Easy Cheese Sauce

Preparation Time:
8 minutes

Serves 8

Serving Size:
1/4 cup

Cheese sauce is a wonderful way to dress up cooked vegetables, but it can be high in fat and calories. Here's a light yet flavorful version you can make in a hurry.

1 1/2 Tbsp all-purpose or unbleached white flour

1/2 tsp dry mustard

1/2 tsp salt, or to taste (optional)

Pinch ground celery seed

1 cup low-fat (1%) milk

1 cup fat-free half-and-half

3–4 drops hot pepper sauce

1 1/4 cups shredded fat-free Cheddar cheese

1. In a small saucepan, stir together the flour, mustard, salt (if desired), and celery seed. Slowly add the milk and half-and-half, stirring with a wire whisk to keep the mixture from lumping. Whisk until the flour is completely incorporated. Add the hot pepper sauce.

2. Over medium heat, cook the milk and flour mixture, whisking until the mixture thickens, about 4 or 5 minutes. Gradually add the cheese, continuing to whisk until the cheese is completely melted.

3. Serve over vegetables such as cooked broccoli, cauliflower, or zucchini.

Exchanges

1/2 Carbohydrate

1 Very Lean Meat

Calories 65

Calories from Fat 7

Total Fat 1 g

Saturated Fat 0.4 g

Cholesterol 5 mg

Sodium 163 mg

Total Carbohydrate 7 g

Dietary Fiber 0 g

Sugars 4 g

Protein 7 g

Preparation Time:
12 minutes

Serves 10

Serving Size:
1/2 cup

Exchanges

1 Starch

Calories 84

Calories from Fat 19

Total Fat 2 g

Saturated Fat 0 g

Cholesterol 0 mg

Sodium 25 mg

Total Carbohydrate
15 g

Dietary Fiber 2 g

Sugars 5 g

Protein 2 g

Roasted Winter Vegetables

Truly delicious, roasted winter vegetables are a great way to add variety to your snacking experience. If you've enjoyed them at a trendy cafe, you'll be glad to know they're a snap to make. Starting the vegetables in the microwave shortens the cooking time considerably.

3 medium onions, cut into large chunks and separated into slices

3 cups red-skinned potatoes, cut into 1-inch pieces

1 1/2 cups baby carrots, cut in half crosswise if the carrots are large

1 medium turnip, peeled and diced

2 Tbsp water

Nonstick cooking spray

1 1/2 Tbsp olive oil

1 garlic clove, minced

1 tsp Italian seasoning

1/2 tsp salt, or to taste (optional)

1/8 tsp black pepper

1. Preheat the oven to 450 degrees. Combine the onions, potatoes, carrots, and turnip in a medium bowl. Add the water.

2. Cover with wax paper and microwave on high power for 6 to 8 minutes, stopping and stirring once, or until the vegetables are partially cooked. Drain the vegetables in a colander.

3. Transfer the vegetables to a large nonstick spray–coated baking pan or rimmed baking sheet. Drizzle with the oil. Sprinkle with the

garlic, Italian seasoning, salt (if desired), and pepper. Stir to mix well.

4. Bake for 30 to 40 minutes, stirring occasionally, or until the vegetables begin to brown and are tender. Serve immediately. Leftover vegetables can be covered and refrigerated for 2 to 3 days and reheated in the microwave.

Pan-Grilled Italian Vegetables

Pan-grilled vegetables make an easy, tasty snack. If you like, substitute chopped cauliflower or broccoli for the zucchini.

1 small onion, coarsely chopped
1 garlic clove, minced
1/4 cup chopped red or green bell pepper
1/4 cup chopped zucchini
1 tsp extra-virgin olive oil
1/4 tsp Italian seasoning
Salt (optional) and pepper to taste

1. In a small nonstick skillet, combine the onion, garlic, red or green pepper, zucchini, and oil. Cook, stirring frequently, over medium heat, until the vegetables are softened and begin to brown slightly.

2. Stir in the Italian seasoning, salt (if desired), and pepper. Serve hot on a 1/2-inch slice of toasted Italian bread or on a small whole-wheat pita bread half.

Exchanges

1 Vegetable

1/2 Fat

Calories 49

Calories from Fat 21

Total Fat 2 g

Saturated Fat 1 g

Cholesterol 0 mg

Sodium 3 mg

Total Carbohydrate 7 g

Dietary Fiber 1 g

Sugars 4 g

Protein 1 g

Israeli Chickpeas

Preparation Time:
3 minutes

Serves 4

Serving Size:
1/2 cup

I've loved chickpeas (garbanzo beans) right from the can since I was a kid, so I was delighted to discover this quick method for making them even better.

Nonstick cooking spray

1 15-oz can chickpeas (garbanzo beans), rinsed and well-drained

1/2 tsp seasoned salt, or to taste (optional), or nonsodium seasoning

Dash black pepper, or to taste

1. Spray a large, heavy nonstick skillet with nonstick cooking spray.

2. Add the chickpeas and season with salt and pepper as desired. Cook over medium heat, shaking skillet often, until the chickpeas are lightly browned, 2 to 4 minutes.

3. Cool slightly before serving. Leftover chickpeas will keep in the refrigerator for 2 to 3 days and can be reheated in the microwave or served cold.

Exchanges

1 Starch

1 Very Lean Meat

Calories 118

Calories from Fat 17

Total Fat 2 g

Saturated Fat 0 g

Cholesterol 0 mg

Sodium 105 mg

Total Carbohydrate 20 g

Dietary Fiber 6 g

Sugars 3 g

Protein 6 g

Preparation Time:
15 minutes

Serves 12

Serving Size:
1/4 cup

Lentils with Cumin and Lemon

I've never met a legume I didn't like, but lentils are one of my favorites. Here's an interesting way to flavor them. Because they're cooked al dente, they still have a bit of crunch. If you prefer, you can cook them to a softer consistency.

1 cup dried brown lentils, washed and sorted
1 small onion, chopped
1 garlic clove, minced
1 celery stalk, minced
2 tsp lemon juice
1 tsp cumin
1/2 tsp salt, or to taste (optional)
1/8 tsp black pepper

Exchanges

1/2 Starch

Calories 54

Calories from Fat 2

Total Fat 0 g

Saturated Fat 0 g

Cholesterol 0 mg

Sodium 4 mg

Total Carbohydrate
10 g

Dietary Fiber 4 g

Sugars 1 g

Protein 4 g

1. In a large saucepan, combine the lentils and 3 cups of water. Cover and bring to a boil. Reduce the heat and simmer for 18 to 20 minutes or until the lentils are tender-crisp. Drain in a colander.

2. In a medium bowl, combine the lentils, onion, garlic, celery, lemon juice, cumin, salt (if desired), and pepper. Stir to mix well.

3. Serve warm, either plain or on fat-free crackers or toasted whole-wheat bread. Or cover and refrigerate until chilled. Lentils will keep in the refrigerator for 3 to 4 days.

Luscious Limas

Preparation Time:
3 minutes

Serves 4

Serving Size:
1/2 cup

Like broccoli, lima beans inspire a strong reaction. If you like them, you'll love this recipe.

1 10-oz package frozen baby lima beans
1 cup frozen mixed pepper and onion stir-fry
2 Tbsp grated Parmesan cheese
1 tsp olive oil
1/8 tsp salt (optional)
Dash black pepper

1. In a medium saucepan over high heat, combine the lima beans, vegetables, and 3/4 cup boiling water. Return to a boil. Cover, lower the heat, and simmer for 12 to 14 minutes or until the beans are tender. Drain in a colander.

2. Transfer the bean mixture to a medium bowl. Stir in the cheese, oil, salt (if desired), and pepper. Serve at once.

3. The beans will keep in the refrigerator for 3 to 4 days.

Exchanges
1/2 Starch
1/2 Fat

Calories 70
Calories from Fat 22
Total Fat 2 g
Saturated Fat 1 g
Cholesterol 4 mg
Sodium 88 mg
Total Carbohydrate 9 g
Dietary Fiber 3 g
Sugars 2 g
Protein 4 g

Crispy Eggplant Sticks with Dipping Sauce

These crispy, oven-baked sticks make an unusual and very tasty snack, especially if you like the flavors of Asian cuisines.

Eggplant sticks:
Nonstick cooking spray

1/3 cup cornmeal

1/3 cup sesame seeds

1/8 tsp each salt and black pepper

1/3 cup liquid egg substitute

1 Tbsp lite soy sauce

1 medium (about 1 lb) eggplant, peeled and cut into 3- by 1-inch sticks

Dipping sauce:
1 small garlic clove, peeled and chopped

1 1/2 tsp peeled and finely minced fresh ginger root

1 1/2 Tbsp lite soy sauce

1 1/2 Tbsp rice vinegar

1 1/2 Tbsp white wine

1 1/2 tsp packed light brown sugar, or to taste

2–4 dashes hot chili oil (optional)

Exchanges

1 Starch

1/2 Fat

Calories 109

Calories from Fat 38

Total Fat 4 g

Saturated Fat 1 g

Cholesterol 0 mg

Sodium 326 mg

Total Carbohydrate
14 g

Dietary Fiber 3 g

Sugars 5 g

Protein 4 g

1. Preheat the oven to 475 degrees. Line a 12- by 18-inch or similar large baking sheet with aluminum foil. Lightly spray with nonstick cooking spray and set aside.

2. In a large shallow bowl, stir together the cornmeal, sesame seeds, salt, and pepper until well mixed. In another bowl, stir together the egg substitute and soy sauce.

3. In batches, dip the eggplant sticks into the egg mixture, removing with a slotted spoon and shaking off any excess. Then toss the eggplant sticks into the cornmeal mixture until evenly coated all over. Lay the sticks, separated, on the baking sheet.

4. Bake in the upper third of the oven until the sticks are nicely browned, about 8 to 10 minutes. Turn over using a spatula.

5. Return to the oven; bake the sticks for 6 to 8 minutes longer, or until well browned and just tender when pierced with a fork. Remove from the oven and set aside.

6. Meanwhile, prepare the dipping sauce by stirring together the garlic, ginger, soy sauce, vinegar, wine, sugar, and chili oil (if desired).

7. Serve warm eggplant sticks with a bowl of dipping sauce on the side. The eggplant and sauce may be covered and kept in the refrigerator for 3 to 4 days. Reheat the eggplant until hot in a 400-degree oven before serving.

Serves 5

Serving Size:
1/2 cup

Exchanges

1 Vegetable

1 Fat

Calories 74

Calories from Fat 52

Total Fat 6 g

Saturated Fat 1 g

Cholesterol 0 mg

Sodium 158 mg

Total Carbohydrate
5 g

Dietary Fiber 2 g

Sugars 3 g

Protein 2 g

Marinated Artichoke Hearts and Cherry Tomatoes

Artichoke hearts and cherry tomatoes complement each other very well. If you like, double this recipe and serve it to a crowd.

2 Tbsp fat-free, low-sodium or regular chicken broth

2 Tbsp olive oil (preferably extra-virgin)

2 Tbsp thinly sliced green onion tops

1 tsp lemon juice

1 tsp apple cider vinegar

1/2 tsp dried thyme leaves

1/2 tsp basil

1/8 tsp salt, or to taste (optional)

1 15-oz can artichoke heart quarters, well drained

1 cup halved cherry tomatoes (15–25, depending on size)

1. In a medium bowl, combine the broth, oil, green onion, lemon juice, vinegar, thyme, basil, and salt (if desired). Stir to mix well.

2. Remove any coarse outer leaves from the artichoke hearts. Stir the artichoke hearts and the tomatoes into the dressing and gently toss to coat.

3. Serve at once, or cover and refrigerate for up to 24 hours. Marinated vegetables will keep in the refrigerator for 3 to 4 days.

Marinated Green Beans

Preparation Time:
15 minutes

Serves 7

Serving Size:
1/2 cup

The tangy sauce perfectly perks up these green beans. I like my beans a little crisp. If you prefer them well done, choose the longer cooking period.

3 1/2 cups (3/4 lb) fresh green beans, trimmed and snapped

2 Tbsp chopped chives or thinly sliced green onion tops

2 Tbsp fat-free, low-sodium, or regular chicken broth or bouillon

1 Tbsp catsup

1 Tbsp balsamic vinegar

2 tsp olive oil

1 tsp Dijon-style mustard

1/4 tsp salt, or to taste (optional)

2–3 drops hot pepper sauce

1. In a large saucepan, cook the beans in boiling water for 10 to 15 minutes until tender-crisp. Drain well in a colander.

2. Meanwhile, in a large bowl, combine the chives, broth, catsup, vinegar, oil, mustard, salt (if desired), and hot pepper sauce. Stir to mix well. Add the cooked beans and stir to coat the beans with marinade.

3. Cover and refrigerate for 2 to 3 hours. Stir before serving. Leftover beans will keep in the refrigerator for 4 to 5 days.

Exchanges
1 Vegetable

Calories 30
Calories from Fat 13
Total Fat 1 g
Saturated Fat 0 g
Cholesterol 0 mg
Sodium 47 mg
Total Carbohydrate 4 g
Dietary Fiber 1 g
Sugars 1 g
Protein 1 g

Stuffed Celery Sticks

If you love the crunch of celery combined with a rich and flavorful filling, try this recipe.

4 oz Neufchâtel cream cheese

1/4 cup low-fat vanilla yogurt

1/2 cup water-packed crushed pineapple, well drained

1/2 cup grated or shredded carrot

2 Tbsp thinly sliced green onion tops

27 5-inch-long celery sticks

1. In a small bowl, stir together the Neufchâtel cheese and yogurt until well combined. Stir in the pineapple, carrot, and onion until well combined.

2. Fill each celery stick with 2 tsp of the mixture. The mixture can be used immediately or covered and refrigerated for up to 24 hours before using. The filling will keep, covered, in the refrigerator for 3 to 4 days.

Exchanges

Free

Calories 18

Calories from Fat 9

Total Fat 1 g

Saturated Fat 1 g

Cholesterol 3 mg

Sodium 35 mg

Total Carbohydrate 2 g

Dietary Fiber 0 g

Sugars 1 g

Protein 1 g

Salad Days

There's nothing like salads for a summer snack. Not only are they tasty, crunchy, and full of flavor, they're good for you, too, because they're packed with vitamins, minerals, and fiber. You'll find a great selection to choose from here. Some are old favorites, like Potato Salad. Others are my own creations, like Pasta, Bean, and Salmon Salad and Turkey Bulgur Salad. Some are simply vegetable combinations. Others add the taste and texture of grains and pasta, like my Carrot-Raisin Salad, which features the flavor and fiber of brown rice. All are made with dressings that are low in fat and calories.

Serves 5

Serving Size:
3/4 cup

Cabbage and Carrot Slaw

This yummy slaw has a great flavor and a pleasing, crunchy texture. And it's a wonderful way to increase your consumption of healthy vegetables. If you like, a small amount of sugar substitute could be used for the sugar in the recipe.

2 Tbsp cider vinegar

2 Tbsp reduced-fat mayonnaise

2 tsp sugar

1/4 tsp dry mustard

1/4 tsp salt, or to taste (optional)

1/8 tsp black pepper

4 cups very thinly sliced cabbage

1 large carrot, grated or shredded

1/2 red bell pepper, seeded and diced

Exchanges

1 Vegetable

1/2 Fat

1. In a large bowl, combine the vinegar, mayonnaise, sugar, mustard, salt (if desired), and black pepper. Whisk until well combined.

2. Add the cabbage, carrot, and pepper. Stir to coat the vegetables with dressing. Serve immediately, or cover and refrigerate. Leftover slaw will keep in the refrigerator for 3 to 4 days.

Calories 51

Calories from Fat 18

Total Fat 2 g

Saturated Fat 0 g

Cholesterol 2 mg

Sodium 51 mg

Total Carbohydrate
8 g

Dietary Fiber 2 g

Sugars 5 g

Protein 1 g

Bean, Corn, and Rice Salad

You'll love the south-of-the-border flavor of this easy, hearty salad. The recipe calls for mild salsa. If you'd like more heat, substitute medium salsa for part of the mild. Brown rice varies considerably in consistency when cooked. Brands that remain firm and separate after cooking work best in this recipe.

3/4 cup mild low-sodium or regular salsa

1 Tbsp olive oil

1/2 tsp dried oregano leaves

1/4 tsp salt, or to taste (optional)

1 15-oz can low-sodium or regular kidney beans, rinsed and well drained

1 cup frozen corn kernels, cooked according to package directions

1 cup cooked brown rice

2 large celery stalks, diced

1. In a medium bowl, combine the salsa, oil, oregano, and salt (if desired). Stir to mix well.

2. Stir in the kidney beans, corn, rice, and celery. Mix well.

3. Serve at once, or cover and refrigerate. Leftover salad will keep in the refrigerator for 3 to 4 days.

Preparation Time: 10 minutes

Serves 9

Serving Size: 1/2 cup

Exchanges

1 Starch

1/2 Fat

Calories 104

Calories from Fat 18

Total Fat 2 g

Saturated Fat 0 g

Cholesterol 0 mg

Sodium 64 mg

Total Carbohydrate 18 g

Dietary Fiber 4 g

Sugars 3 g

Protein 4 g

Broccoli-Rice Salad

Here's a tasty way to enjoy broccoli. The recipe works best when made with a mild-flavored brown rice that holds its shape well after cooking.

4 cups small broccoli florets

3 Tbsp reduced-fat mayonnaise

1/4 cup low-fat buttermilk

2 tsp cider vinegar

1 tsp sugar

1/8 tsp ground celery seed

1/8 tsp white pepper

1/8 tsp salt, or to taste (optional)

1 cup cooked brown rice

2 Tbsp chopped red onion

Exchanges

1/2 Starch

1 Vegetable

1/2 Fat

Calories 71

Calories from Fat 22

Total Fat 2 g

Saturated Fat 0 g

Cholesterol 3 mg

Sodium 60 mg

Total Carbohydrate
11 g

Dietary Fiber 2 g

Sugars 3 g

Protein 2 g

1. To bring out the bright green color of the broccoli, place it in a medium saucepan with 1/4 cup water. Bring to a boil and then boil for 1 minute. Remove from heat and cool in a colander under cold running water. Drain.

2. Place the mayonnaise in a large serving bowl. Slowly add the buttermilk, whisking until smooth. Whisk in the vinegar, sugar, celery seed, pepper, and salt (if desired). Stir in the rice, reserved broccoli, and onion.

3. Serve at room temperature, or cover and refrigerate for several hours. Leftover salad will keep in the refrigerator for 2 to 3 days. Stir before serving.

Carrot-Raisin Salad

Preparation Time:
12 minutes

Serves 4

Serving Size:
1/2 cup

If you like the crunch and tang of traditional carrot-raisin salad, you'll love this version. The recipe calls for a teaspoon of optional honey, which enhances the sweetness of the carrots. But you could leave it out if you like.

2 Tbsp reduced-fat mayonnaise

1/4 cup low-fat buttermilk

1/2 Tbsp cider vinegar

1 tsp mild or strong honey (optional)

1 cup cooked brown rice

3 medium carrots, grated or shredded (1 cup)

1/3 cup dark raisins

1. Place the mayonnaise in a medium bowl. Slowly add the buttermilk, whisking until well combined. Whisk in the vinegar and honey (if desired).

2. Add the rice, carrots, and raisins, and stir to mix well.

3. Serve at once, or cover and refrigerate for several hours before serving. Leftover salad will keep in the refrigerator for 3 to 4 days.

Exchanges

1 Starch

1 Fruit

Calories 143

Calories from Fat 27

Total Fat 3 g

Saturated Fat 1 g

Cholesterol 4 mg

Sodium 76 mg

Total Carbohydrate 28 g

Dietary Fiber 2 g

Sugars 13 g

Protein 3 g

Cajun Rice and Bean Salad

Preparation Time:
12 minutes

Serves 10

Serving Size:
1/2 cup

Here's a spicy New Orleans–style rice and bean salad. For best results, use brown rice that retains its shape after cooking.

1 cup low-sodium or regular stewed tomatoes

1 Tbsp olive oil

1/2 Tbsp cider vinegar

1/2 tsp dried marjoram leaves

1/2 tsp dried thyme leaves

1/4 tsp salt, or to taste (optional)

2–3 drops hot pepper sauce

2 cups cooked brown rice

1 15-oz can low-sodium or regular kidney beans, rinsed and well drained

1/4 cup thinly sliced green onion, including tops

1 large celery stalk, diced

1. In a medium bowl, combine the tomatoes, oil, vinegar, marjoram, thyme, salt (if desired), and hot pepper sauce. Stir to mix well.

2. Stir in the rice, beans, onion, and celery.

3. Serve the salad at room temperature, or cover and refrigerate before serving. Leftover salad will keep in the refrigerator for 2 to 3 days.

Exchanges

1 Starch

1/2 Fat

Calories 100

Calories from Fat 17

Total Fat 2 g

Saturated Fat 0 g

Cholesterol 0 mg

Sodium 16 mg

Total Carbohydrate 17 g

Dietary Fiber 3 g

Sugars 2 g

Protein 4 g

Spanish Rice Salad

Preparation Time:
10 minutes

Serves 6

Serving Size:
1/2 cup

If you enjoy Spanish rice, try this salad variation.

2 cups cooked brown rice (about 1/2 cup uncooked)

1 Tbsp olive oil

1/2 Tbsp lemon juice

1 medium tomato, diced

1/2 sweet red pepper, seeded and diced

1/4 cup thinly sliced green onion, including tops

1/4 cup chopped fresh parsley

1 garlic clove, minced

1/4 tsp salt, or to taste (optional)

1. In a medium bowl, stir together the rice, olive oil, and lemon juice.

2. Stir in the tomato, pepper, onion, parsley, garlic, and salt (if desired). Mix well. Serve at room temperature, or cover and refrigerate for several hours.

3. Leftover salad will keep in the refrigerator, covered, for 3 to 4 days.

Exchanges

1 Starch

1/2 Fat

Calories 105

Calories from Fat 27

Total Fat 3 g

Saturated Fat 1 g

Cholesterol 0 mg

Sodium 8 mg

Total Carbohydrate 18 g

Dietary Fiber 2 g

Sugars 2 g

Protein 2 g

Preparation Time:
12 minutes

Serves 4

Serving Size:
1/2 cup

The Chinese noodles called for in this recipe are the curly variety, similar to ramen noodles. They're available in specialty food markets and many grocery stores.

1/3 10-oz package Chinese noodles

1/4 cup fat-free, low-sodium or regular chicken broth

1 Tbsp smooth peanut butter

2 tsp light soy sauce

2 tsp Asian sesame oil

1 1/2 tsp rice or white vinegar

1/2 tsp ginger

3–4 drops hot pepper sauce

1/2 cup peeled and chopped broccoli stems

2 Tbsp chopped chives or sliced green onions

1. Cook the noodles according to the package directions. Rinse under cold water and drain in a colander. When the noodles are well drained, transfer to a medium bowl. Cut or tear long strands into smaller pieces.

2. In a small deep microwave-safe bowl, combine the broth, peanut butter, soy sauce, oil, vinegar, ginger, and hot pepper sauce. Microwave for 20 to 30 seconds to warm the mixture so that the peanut butter will easily combine with the other ingredients. With a small wire whisk, whisk until well combined. Stir in the broccoli and chives.

3. Stir the dressing mixture into the noodles. Serve warm, or cover and refrigerate. Leftover noodle salad will keep in the refrigerator for 3 to 4 days.

Exchanges

1 1/2 Starch

1/2 Fat

Calories 135

Calories from Fat 51

Total Fat 6 g

Saturated Fat 1 g

Cholesterol 0 mg

Sodium 253 mg

Total Carbohydrate 21 g

Dietary Fiber 1 g

Sugars 2 g

Protein 4 g

Pasta, Bean, and Salmon Salad

Quick and easy, this delicious salad can be made from ingredients that are probably in your pantry, and you can make the dressing and finish the rest of the preparations while the pasta is cooking.

3 Tbsp catsup

2 Tbsp cider vinegar

1 Tbsp olive oil

1 garlic clove, minced

1 tsp Italian seasoning

1/8 tsp salt, or to taste (optional)

1 cup uncooked penne or similarly shaped pasta

1 14 1/2-oz can low-sodium cut green beans, well drained

2 Tbsp chopped red onion or other sweet onion

1 6-oz can boneless, skinless pink salmon, well drained

1. In a large serving bowl, combine the catsup and vinegar. Stir to mix well. Stir in the oil, garlic, Italian seasoning, and salt (if desired). Set aside.

2. Cook the pasta according to package directions. Transfer to a colander and rinse under cold running water. Drain.

3. Meanwhile, add the green beans and onion to the bowl with the dressing. Stir to mix well. Stir in the pasta and salmon.

4. Serve immediately, or cover and refrigerate for 1 hour or up to 36 hours before serving. Stir before serving. Leftover salad will keep in the refrigerator for 3 to 4 days.

Exchanges
1/2 Starch
1 Lean Meat

Calories 100

Calories from Fat 28

Total Fat 3 g

Saturated Fat 0 g

Cholesterol 12 mg

Sodium 190 mg

Total Carbohydrate 12 g

Dietary Fiber 1 g

Sugars 2 g

Protein 6 g

Marinated Potato Salad

Potatoes that are just a little bit crisp work best in this zesty salad, since they hold together well when stirred into the dressing.

5 medium (about 1 1/2 lb) red-skinned potatoes, cut into 1/2-inch cubes

3 Tbsp fat-free, low-sodium or regular chicken broth

2 Tbsp olive oil

1 1/2 Tbsp plus 1 tsp balsamic vinegar

1 large celery stalk, thinly sliced

3 Tbsp chopped red onion or other sweet onion

1 1/2 tsp Dijon-style mustard

3/4 tsp basil

3/4 tsp dried thyme leaves

1/4 tsp salt, or to taste (optional)

2–3 drops hot pepper sauce

Exchanges

1 Starch

Calories 81

Calories from Fat 25

Total Fat 3 g

Saturated Fat 1 g

Cholesterol 0 mg

Sodium 31 mg

Total Carbohydrate 13 g

Dietary Fiber 2 g

Sugars 2 g

Protein 2 g

1. Combine the potatoes and enough water to cover in a large saucepan. Cover the pot and bring to a boil over high heat. Reduce the heat and simmer for 6 to 11 minutes, until the potatoes are tender but not soft when pierced with a fork. Cool under cold running water. Drain well in a colander.

2. While the potatoes are cooking, in a large bowl or serving dish, combine the broth, oil, and vinegar. Stir to mix. Add the celery, onion, mustard, basil, thyme, salt (if desired), and hot pepper sauce. Stir to mix well.

3. To assemble the salad, add the potatoes, carefully stirring with a large spoon to coat them with the dressing mixture. Be careful not to break up the potatoes. Cover and refrigerate for several hours, stirring occasionally, to allow the flavors to blend. Leftover salad will keep for 3 to 4 days in the refrigerator.

Potato Salad

This potato salad has a tasty ranch-style dressing that combines reduced-fat mayonnaise and low-fat buttermilk. A number of steps will help you prepare this snack quickly. Cut up the potatoes before cooking them, and have the boiling water ready. Mix the dressing while the potatoes are cooking, and cool them quickly under cold running water.

5 cups (about 1 1/2 lb) red-skinned potatoes,
    cut into 3/4-inch cubes

1/4 cup reduced-fat mayonnaise

1/2 cup low-fat buttermilk

3/4 tsp basil

3/4 tsp dried thyme leaves

3/4 tsp dried marjoram leaves

1/8 tsp celery seed

1/4 tsp salt, or to taste (optional)

2–3 drops hot pepper sauce

1 small cucumber, peeled, seeded, and cubed

2 Tbsp chopped chives or green onions

Exchanges

1 Starch

Calories 68

Calories from Fat 15

Total Fat 2 g

Saturated Fat 0 g

Cholesterol 2 mg

Sodium 45 mg

Total Carbohydrate
12 g

Dietary Fiber 1 g

Sugars 2 g

Protein 2 g

1. In a small pot or very large saucepan, combine the potatoes with 1 quart of boiling water. Cover and bring to a boil again. Reduce the heat and boil for 9 to 14 minutes. Do not overcook. Cool in a colander under cold running water. Drain well.

2. Meanwhile, place the mayonnaise in a large serving bowl. Slowly add the buttermilk, whisking until smooth. Stir in the basil, thyme, marjoram, celery seed, salt (if desired), and hot

pepper sauce. Stir in the cucumber and chives. Gently stir in the cooled and drained potatoes.

3. Serve warm, or cover and refrigerate for 1 or 2 hours, or cool in the freezer for 15 to 20 minutes. Cover and refrigerate. Leftover salad will keep in the refrigerator for 3 to 4 days.

Preparation Time:
18 minutes

Serves 16

Serving Size:
1/2 cup

Pasta-Vegetable Salad

If summer tomatoes are unavailable, substitute 5 or 6 Italian plum tomatoes. If you like, a small amount of sugar substitute could be used in place of the sugar in the recipe.

2 Tbsp cider vinegar

2 Tbsp tomato sauce

2 tsp sugar

2 Tbsp olive oil

1 garlic clove, minced

1/4 tsp dried marjoram leaves

1/4 tsp basil

1/4 tsp salt, or to taste (optional)

1 cup uncooked penne or similarly shaped pasta

1 large tomato, cubed

1 small zucchini, cubed

1 medium red or yellow pepper, seeded and chopped

1 cup broccoli or cauliflower florets

Exchanges

1/2 Starch

Calories 44

Calories from Fat 17

Total Fat 2 g

Saturated Fat 0 g

Cholesterol 0 mg

Sodium 14 mg

Total Carbohydrate
6 g

Dietary Fiber 1 g

Sugars 2 g

Protein 1 g

1. In a serving bowl, combine the vinegar and tomato sauce. Stir to mix well. Stir in the sugar, oil, garlic, marjoram, basil, and salt (if desired). Set aside.

2. Cook the pasta according to package directions. Transfer to a colander and rinse under cold running water. Drain.

3. Meanwhile, add the tomatoes, zucchini, pepper, and broccoli to the bowl with the dressing. Stir to mix well. Stir in pasta. Serve immediately, or cover and refrigerate for 1 hour or up to 36 hours before serving. Stir before serving.

Three-Bean Snack

Preparation Time:
10 minutes

Serves 8

Serving Size:
1/2 cup

Try this quick and easy variation of the popular three-bean salad.

1/4 cup chili sauce

3 Tbsp fat-free, low-sodium or regular chicken broth

1 1/2 Tbsp red wine vinegar

1 Tbsp olive oil

2 tsp Italian seasoning

2–3 drops hot pepper sauce

1/4 tsp salt, or to taste (optional)

1 16-oz can low-sodium or regular kidney beans, rinsed and well drained

1 14 1/2-oz can wax beans, rinsed and well drained

1 14 1/2-oz can low-sodium or regular cut green beans, rinsed and well drained

2 Tbsp chopped red onion or other sweet onion

1. In a large bowl, combine the chili sauce, broth, vinegar, oil, Italian seasoning, hot pepper sauce, and salt (if desired). Stir to mix well.

2. Add the beans and onion and stir gently to coat with the dressing.

3. Serve at once or cover and refrigerate. Leftover salad will keep in the refrigerator for 3 to 4 days.

Exchanges

1/2 Starch

1 Vegetable

1/2 Fat

Calories 80

Calories from Fat 17

Total Fat 2 g

Saturated Fat 0 g

Cholesterol 0 mg

Sodium 260 mg

Total Carbohydrate 12 g

Dietary Fiber 4 g

Sugars 3 g

Protein 4 g

Preparation Time:
11 minutes

Serves 9

Serving Size:
1/2 cup

Italian Bread Salad

The Italians invented this chunky salad as a way to use up stale bread. I prefer lightly toasted whole-wheat bread cut into cubes.

3 Tbsp fat-free, low-sodium or regular chicken broth

2 Tbsp grated Parmesan cheese

1 1/2 Tbsp olive oil

1 Tbsp red wine vinegar

1/8 tsp salt (optional)

1/8 tsp black pepper

1 1/2 cups (about 15–25) cherry tomatoes, sliced in half before measuring

1 medium cucumber, peeled, seeded, and cubed

2 Tbsp thinly sliced chives or green onion tops

2 Tbsp chopped fresh basil leaves or 1/4 tsp dried basil leaves

2 cups 1/2-inch bread cubes

Exchanges

1/2 Starch

1/2 Fat

Calories 63

Calories from Fat 30

Total Fat 3 g

Saturated Fat 1 g

Cholesterol 2 mg

Sodium 102 mg

Total Carbohydrate 7 g

Dietary Fiber 1 g

Sugars 2 g

Protein 2 g

1. In a 2-cup measure or similar deep bowl, combine the broth, cheese, oil, vinegar, salt (if desired), and pepper. Stir briskly with a fork to mix well. Set aside.

2. In a medium salad bowl, mix together the tomato, cucumber, chives, and fresh basil. (If using dried basil, mix it into the salad dressing.)

3. Pour the dressing over the vegetables and toss to mix. Add the bread cubes and thoroughly toss to coat them with dressing. Serve at once. This salad will keep for a day in the refrigerator, although the bread tends to absorb the dressing.

Tabouli

This traditional Middle Eastern salad is filling and flavorful.

1 cup dry bulgur wheat

1 1/2 cups boiling water

2 Tbsp lemon juice

2 Tbsp olive oil

2 garlic cloves, minced

1 tsp salt, or to taste (optional)

2–3 drops hot pepper sauce (optional)

1/4 cup sliced green onion tops

2 Tbsp fresh mint leaves or 1/2 tsp dried mint

1/2 cup coarsely chopped fresh parsley

1 large tomato, diced

1 small cucumber, peeled, seeded, and diced

1. In a large bowl, combine the bulgur and boiling water. Cover and let stand for 15 to 20 minutes, until the bulgur has softened and most of the water has been absorbed. Drain in a sieve. Return the bulgur to the bowl.

2. Add the lemon juice, oil, garlic, salt (if desired), and hot pepper sauce (if desired). Stir to mix well. Stir in the onions, mint, parsley, tomato, and cucumber. Stir the vegetable mixture into the bulgur.

3. Serve at once, or cover and refrigerate for several hours. Stir before serving. Leftover tabouli will keep in the refrigerator for 2 to 3 days.

Preparation Time:
30 minutes

Serves 6

Serving Size:
1/2 cup

Exchanges

1 Starch

1 Vegetable

1/2 Fat

Calories 135

Calories from Fat 45

Total Fat 5 g

Saturated Fat 1 g

Cholesterol 0 mg

Sodium 12 mg

Total Carbohydrate 21 g

Dietary Fiber 5 g

Sugars 2 g

Protein 4 g

Preparation Time:
30 minutes

Serves 4

Serving Size:
1/2 cup

Exchanges

1 Starch

1 Lean Meat

Calories 127

Calories from Fat 34

Total Fat 4 g

Saturated Fat 1 g

Cholesterol 17 mg

Sodium 48 mg

Total Carbohydrate
15 g

Dietary Fiber 4 g

Sugars 1 g

Protein 9 g

Turkey Bulgur Salad

1/2 cup bulgur wheat

1 cup boiling water

2 Tbsp fat-free, low-sodium or regular chicken broth

1 Tbsp olive oil

1/2 Tbsp lemon juice

1/2 tsp dried thyme leaves

1/2 tsp dry mustard

3/4 cup (3 oz) cooked turkey breast, cut into small pieces

1 celery stalk, chopped

1/4 cup red bell pepper, seeded and chopped

2 Tbsp chopped fresh parsley

2 Tbsp red onion, minced

1/4 tsp salt, or to taste (optional)

Dash black pepper

1. In a medium bowl, combine the bulgur and boiling water. Cover and let stand for 15 to 20 minutes, until the bulgur has softened and most of the water has been absorbed. Drain in a sieve. Return the bulgur to the bowl.

2. While the bulgur is softening, in a medium bowl, combine the broth, oil, lemon juice, thyme, and dry mustard. Stir to mix well.

3. Stir in the turkey, celery, red pepper, parsley, onion, salt (if desired), and pepper.

4. Stir the turkey mixture into the softened bulgur. Serve at once, or cover and refrigerate for several hours. Stir before serving. Leftover salad will keep in the refrigerator for 2 to 3 days.

Turkey Salad with Apples and Almonds

You'll love this variation of a classic chicken salad! This recipe calls for toasting the almonds, which adds wonderful flavor to the salad.

Nonstick cooking spray

2 Tbsp sliced almonds

3 Tbsp fat-free sour cream

1 Tbsp reduced-fat mayonnaise

Dash ground celery seed

Dash ground cardamom

1/8 tsp salt or to taste (optional)

1 cup (5 oz) roasted turkey or chicken breast cubes

1 cup cubed tart or sweet apple, peeled or unpeeled

1 small celery stalk, diced

1. Spray a medium nonstick skillet with nonstick spray. Add the almonds. Over medium heat, cook the almonds, stirring, until they brown and smell toasted, about 4 or 5 minutes. If the almonds begin to burn, lower the heat slightly. Immediately remove to a small plate and set aside.

2. In a medium bowl, stir together the sour cream, mayonnaise, celery seed, cardamom, and salt (if desired).

3. Stir in the turkey, apple, celery, and reserved almonds. Serve at once, or cover and refrigerate for several hours or up to 24 hours. Leftover salad will keep in the refrigerator for 2 to 3 days.

Preparation Time:
16 minutes

Serves 4

Serving Size:
1/2 cup

Exchanges
1/2 Carbohydrate
1 Lean Meat

Calories 111
Calories from Fat 30
Total Fat 3 g
Saturated Fat 0 g
Cholesterol 30 mg
Sodium 78 mg
Total Carbohydrate 8 g
Dietary Fiber 2 g
Sugars 6 g
Protein 12 g

Curried Turkey Salad

Curry and pineapple make a wonderful foil for the turkey breast meat in this salad. You can buy a turkey breast and roast it at home, reserving the remaining meat for another purpose. Or you can buy thick-cut roasted turkey breast from a deli or a package of roasted turkey breast meat.

1/2 cup juice-packed crushed pineapple, well drained

1/4 cup fat-free sour cream

2 Tbsp reduced-fat mayonnaise

1 tsp mild curry powder

1/4 tsp salt, or to taste (optional)

1 cup (5 oz) cubed turkey breast meat

1 8-oz can sliced water chestnuts, well drained

1 small celery stalk, chopped

2 Tbsp chopped chives or sliced green onion tops

1. In a medium bowl, stir together the pineapple, sour cream, mayonnaise, curry powder, and salt (if desired).

2. Stir in the turkey, water chestnuts, celery, and chives. Serve at once, or cover and refrigerate for several hours or up to 24 hours. Leftover salad will keep in the refrigerator for 2 to 3 days.

Exchanges

1/2 Fruit

1 Vegetable

1 Very Lean Meat

Calories 97

Calories from Fat 19

Total Fat 2 g

Saturated Fat 0 g

Cholesterol 25 mg

Sodium 89 mg

Total Carbohydrate 10 g

Dietary Fiber 1 g

Sugars 6 g

Protein 10 g

Just for Kids

The recipes in this chapter are fun to make and fun to munch! Many, like my Pear Mice, Celery Man, and Alphabet Letters, are designed to get little kids interested in eating the fruits and vegetables that are so good for them. Others are fanciful interpretations of the sandwich theme. And there are two sweet and crunchy popcorn snacks that go easy on the syrup.

While these recipes are designed especially for kids, there are a lot of others elsewhere in this book, like my Egg 'n' Muffin, Quick Turkey Salad Sandwich, or Pizza Puffs, that make great after-school snacks. Other kid pleasers include Easy Cheese Popcorn, Cranberry-Orange Muffins, and Carrot-Raisin Salad.

On the other hand, my adult friends have enjoyed many of the recipes in this chapter, too. So don't think you have to be a kid to try snacks like French Toast Bites, Cinnamon Triangles, Caramel Apples, or a Banana Pop.

Preparation Time:
10 minutes

Serves 1

Celery Man

Here's a whimsical vegetable man who's fun to eat.

1 large celery stalk with some leaves, if possible

2 raisins

1 dried cranberry

1 Tbsp cottage cheese spread (see recipe, p. 5), plain low-fat cottage cheese, flavored fat-free yogurt, or canned shredded beets

1. To make the man, lay a large celery stalk on a flat surface with the leafy part facing away from you and the concave side up. The leaves and stem pieces above the joint will be the hair. The next inch of stalk will be the head.

2. To make the head stand out from the body, create a neck by carving two shallow half-moon shapes into the sides of the stalk. For the arms, carefully cut two long slivers at the sides of the stalk below the neck. Gently pull the arms to a 45-degree angle from the body, being careful not to detach them.

3. For the legs, make a 3- or 4-inch cut from the bottom of the stalk toward the top. Gently open the legs slightly, being careful not to detach them.

4. To make the face, use two raisins for eyes and a dried cranberry for a mouth. Dress the body of the man by spooning on 1 Tbsp of desired spread or topping.

Exchanges

1 Vegetable

Calories 29

Calories from Fat 3

Total Fat 0 g

Saturated Fat 0 g

Cholesterol 1 mg

Sodium 109 mg

Total Carbohydrate 4 g

Dietary Fiber 1 g

Sugars 3 g

Protein 2 g

Pear Mice

Preparation Time:
6 minutes

Serves 1

Here's a fun way to enjoy pear salad—turn pear halves into cute little mice. The recipe gives one garnishing suggestion. But you could also use cut strawberries for ears, a piece of cooked pasta for a tail, and a raisin for a nose.

2 juice-packed canned pear halves

1 dried cranberry, cut in half

4 currants (or 2 dark raisins cut in half and rounded)

2 grapes, cut in half lengthwise (or two golden raisins, flattened)

2 3-inch slivers of sweet pepper or celery

1. Lay the pear halves, cut side down, on a plate. You can position both pieces with the narrow end facing either toward you or away from you, or one of each. The narrow end of the pear will be the face and the big end will be the body.

2. To turn a pear half into a mouse, lay half a dried cranberry at the tip of the narrow end for a nose. Press two currants into place above the nose for eyes. Make the ears of grape halves, set in place on either side of the head. If necessary, cut small slits in the pear flesh to hold the ears erect.

3. To make the tail, lay a sliver of sweet pepper or celery at the large end of the mouse. Repeat with the second pear half.

Exchanges
1 1/2 Fruit

Calories 77
Calories from Fat 2
Total Fat 0 g
Saturated Fat 0 g
Cholesterol 0 mg
Sodium 5 mg
Total Carbohydrate 20 g
Dietary Fiber 3 g
Sugars 15 g
Protein 1 g

Mr. and Mrs. Pear Head

Mr. and Mrs. Pear Head are a fun addition to afternoon snack time. You can use a variety of fruit and vegetable pieces to make the eyes, nose, mouth, and hair. Below are several suggestions, but you could also use a cut piece of strawberry for the mouth, red grapes for eyes, and currants or pieces of dried apricot for various features. For variety, try shredded lettuce or shoe-string beets for hair. Either the narrow end or the wide end of the pear can be the top of the head.

2 juice-packed canned pear halves

4 raisins

2 carrot half circles

1/4 cup grated carrot or crushed pineapple

Exchanges

1 Fruit

1 Vegetable

Calories 85

Calories from Fat 2

Total Fat 0 g

Saturated Fat 0 g

Cholesterol 0 mg

Sodium 19 mg

Total Carbohydrate
22 g

Dietary Fiber 4 g

Sugars 16 g

Protein 1 g

1. Lay the pear halves, cut side down, on a plate.

2. Give the pear halves eyes and mouths. Use two raisins for eyes on each pair half and press them into place. Place the carrot half circles into place for the mouths.

3. For hair, arrange grated carrot or crushed pineapple on the plate at the top of the head. Or give Mrs. Pear Head all the hair and leave her husband bald.

Dugout Canoes

Preparation Time:
6 minutes

Serves 2

Serving Size: 1
canoe

It's fun to remove the seeds from a cucumber and fill the cavity with vegetable stick logs. Or fill with Tuna Salad (p. 12), Salmon Salad (p. 11), Quick Turkey Salad (p. 39), or Cottage Cheese with Dill and Onion (p. 5; the nutritional analysis was calculated using this filling).

1 medium cucumber

1 carrot, cut into sticks

1 celery stalk, cut into 2-inch sections

1 Tbsp filling of choice (optional, see suggestions above)

1. With a vegetable peeler, remove the skin from the cucumber. Lay the cucumber on a flat surface and cut in half lengthwise.

2. With a teaspoon, carefully scrape the seeds from the cucumber and discard them.

3. Fill with carrot and celery sticks or filling of choice.

Exchanges
1 Vegetable

Calories 30

Calories from Fat 4

Total Fat 0 g

Saturated Fat 0 g

Cholesterol 1 mg

Sodium 88 mg

Total Carbohydrate 3 g

Dietary Fiber 2 g

Sugars 4 g

Protein 2 g

Mad Teacup

This fruit cup was inspired by the mad spinning teacup rides we've all enjoyed at many amusement parks. If you want to re-create the whirling motion by spinning your plate, do it carefully!

1/2 medium apple, cored
1/2 tsp lemon juice
1 juice-packed pineapple ring
1/4 cup berries or diced fruit
Mint sprig (optional)

1. With a teaspoon or small knife, carefully dig out some of the apple flesh so that the half apple forms a cup. Rub the lemon juice over the apple surface.

2. Place the pineapple ring on a small plate. Set the apple in the center of the ring. Fill the apple center with berries or diced fruit. Garnish with a sprig of mint, if you like.

Exchanges

1 Fruit

Calories 73

Calories from Fat 4

Total Fat 0 g

Saturated Fat 0 g

Cholesterol 0 mg

Sodium 1 mg

Total Carbohydrate
19 g

Dietary Fiber 3 g

Sugars 15 g

Protein 0 g

Egg Sailboats

Preparation Time:
3 minutes

Serves 1

These cute little egg sailboats skim across the plate. (In fact, it would be fun to serve them on a blue paper plate.) The yolks are removed and replaced with a healthier filling, such as Tuna Salad (p. 12; the nutritional analysis was calculated using this filling), Quick Turkey Salad (p. 39), or the Better Deviled Eggs mixture (p. 43). Use a triangle cut from a cabbage leaf, a sweet pepper, or a piece of spinach for the sail. Or, for an interesting variation, omit the sail and fill the cavity with Guacamole (p. 9) or mashed green peas and call them "green eggs." You could even serve them with a thin slice of low-fat deli ham!

1 hard-cooked large egg

1 Tbsp filling of choice (see suggestions above)

1 2-inch-high triangle cut from a cabbage or spinach leaf or a piece of sweet pepper

1. Cut the egg in half and scoop out and discard the yolk. Fill the cavity with filling of choice.

2. Stick a vegetable triangle into the top of the filling to serve as a sail for the egg boat.

Exchanges

1 Very Lean Meat

Calories 41

Calories from Fat 8

Total Fat 1 g

Saturated Fat 0 g

Cholesterol 5 mg

Sodium 114 mg

Total Carbohydrate 1 g

Dietary Fiber 0 g

Sugars 1 g

Protein 7 g

Alphabet Letters

Preparation Time:
15 minutes

Serves 2

Serving Size:
1 cup

How many letters of the alphabet can you make from vegetable pieces? How many words? It's fun to find out! Straight pieces cut from vegetables like celery, carrot, zucchini, and green beans can form many letters, such as A, T, E, F, and H. Carrot, zucchini, and cucumber circles and half circles make the curves of letters like B, C, D, and O. Use a colorful mixture of vegetables to create letters and words.

30 straight vegetable pieces, about 2 inches long and 1/4 inch wide, cut from celery, carrot, cucumber, zucchini, red pepper, green pepper, and green beans

20 vegetable circles and half circles cut from carrot, cucumber, zucchini, and yellow squash

2 Tbsp reduced-fat salad dressing

1. Serve the vegetable pieces on two separate plates—one for straight pieces and one for rounds. Select from the pieces to make letters of the alphabet and words.

2. Decorate the finished letters and words with salad dressing and eat!

Exchanges

1 Vegetable

1/2 Fat

Calories 42

Calories from Fat 16

Total Fat 2 g

Saturated Fat 0 g

Cholesterol 0 mg

Sodium 116 mg

Total Carbohydrate 9 g

Dietary Fiber 3 g

Sugars 5 g

Protein 1 g

Vegetable Centipede

Preparation Time:
12 minutes

Serves 1

Make raw vegetables into a creepy, crawly critter with this fun-to-eat centipede. You can also use a broccoli or cauliflower floret or a large radish for the critter's head and zucchini or yellow squash rounds for the body. Try cutting orange eyes from a piece of carrot or red eyes from a sweet red pepper. It works best to pick contrasting colors for the body and the legs.

7 carrot, cucumber, or cooked beet circles

12 celery or carrot sticks, about 2 inches long and 1/3 inch wide

2 fresh or frozen green peas

2 thin celery pieces

1 green onion, root trimmed so that about an inch of green top is left attached to the white part

1 Tbsp reduced-fat salad dressing

1. On a large plate, lay the circle pieces in a line, one behind the other to form the body of the centipede, curving the line slightly, if desired. Use the largest circle for the head at the top of the line. Arrange the celery or carrot sticks so that they stick out at right angles on either side of the body segments to form legs. (There will be no legs on the head segment.)

2. Arrange two peas on the head segment for eyes. Position two thin celery pieces for antennae. Make vertical cuts in the green top of the onion to create a brush-like effect. Fan out the brush to form a tail, and lay it below the last segment. Let the snacker decorate the centipede with salad dressing.

Exchanges
1 Vegetable
1/2 Fat

Calories 56
Calories from Fat 28
Total Fat 3 g
Saturated Fat 1 g
Cholesterol 4 mg
Sodium 134 mg
Total Carbohydrate 6 g
Dietary Fiber 2 g
Sugars 3 g
Protein 1 g

Serves 10

Serving Size:
  1 cup

Easy Caramel Popcorn

The directions call for finishing this easy popcorn snack by baking it to harden the syrup. If you don't mind sticky popcorn, you can skip the baking step. In any case, be sure to cool the popcorn before serving, as hot syrup can burn your mouth.

Nonstick cooking spray
10 cups popped low-fat microwave popcorn
6 caramel candies, cut into small pieces
2 Tbsp dark or light corn syrup
1/2 Tbsp water

1. Preheat the oven to 350 degrees. Spray a large jelly roll pan or rimmed cookie sheet with nonstick cooking spray and set aside. Place the popcorn in a large ceramic or glass bowl and set aside.

2. In a 1-cup measure or similar microwave-safe bowl, combine the caramels, syrup, and water. Cover with wax paper and microwave on high power for 40 seconds. Stir. Microwave for an additional 30 seconds until the caramels are completely melted.

3. Being very careful to keep fingers away from the hot syrup, slowly pour the caramel mixture over the popcorn, stirring with a large wooden spoon to coat evenly. Spread the popcorn evenly on the prepared baking pan. Bake the popcorn for 4 to 6 minutes until the syrup hardens slightly.

4. Cool before serving, or store tightly covered at room temperature. Leftover popcorn will keep for 4 to 5 days.

Exchanges

1/2 Carbohydrate

Calories 53

Calories from Fat 7

Total Fat 1 g

Saturated Fat 0 g

Cholesterol 1 mg

Sodium 59 mg

Total Carbohydrate
  11 g

Dietary Fiber 1 g

Sugars 6 g

Protein 1 g

Popcorn Crunch

Preparation Time:
20 minutes

Serves 10

Serving Size: 1 cup

Coating popcorn with syrup is a great way to satisfy a sweet tooth, since it makes a little syrup go a long way. Check nutritional labels on microwave popcorn, as some brands have more fat than others.

Nonstick cooking spray

10 cups popped low-fat microwave popcorn

1/3 cup sugar

3 Tbsp molasses

1 Tbsp water

1 tsp vanilla extract

1. Spray a very large (at least 10 1/2- by 13 1/2- inch) baking pan with nonstick spray. Set aside. Preheat the oven to 375 degrees. Remove and discard un- popped kernels from popcorn. Set popcorn aside.

2. In a small saucepan, combine the sugar, molasses, and water and stir to mix well. Cook over medium- high heat, stirring with a wooden spoon, until the mixture comes to a full boil. Boil, stirring constantly, for 1 minute.

3. Remove from heat. With a wooden spoon, stir in vanilla until completely combined. Slowly drizzle the syrup over the popcorn, stirring well to coat evenly and keeping fingers away from hot syrup.

4. Spread the popcorn evenly in the pan. Bake on center oven rack for 5 to 6 minutes until the pop- corn begins to crisp slightly. Remove from the oven and stir. Cool. Syrup will harden and popcorn will crisp further as it cools. When cool, store in a sealed plastic bag or airtight container for 2 to 3 days.

Exchanges

1 Carbohydrate

Calories 72

Calories from Fat 7

Total Fat 1 g

Saturated Fat 0 g

Cholesterol 0 mg

Sodium 3 mg

Total Carbohydrate 17 g

Dietary Fiber 1 g

Sugars 10 g

Protein 1 g

Caramel Apples

Caramel and apple make a great combination! This easy variation calls for cored apple cut into pieces and stirred into the syrup. An added advantage is that you can make this recipe with very little candy.

2 1/2 caramel candies, cut into small pieces
1/2 Tbsp dark or light corn syrup
1 large tart apple, cored and cut into bite-sized
    pieces

1. In a 1-cup measure or similar microwave-safe bowl, combine the caramels and corn syrup. Microwave on high power for 30 seconds. Stir and microwave for 15 additional seconds, or until the caramels are completely melted.

2. Stir well, and mix in the apple pieces, stirring to coat them with syrup. Cool slightly. Divide into two servings. Eat with a fork.

Exchanges

2 Carbohydrate

Calories 120

Calories from Fat 11

Total Fat 1 g

Saturated Fat 1 g

Cholesterol 1 mg

Sodium 35 mg

Total Carbohydrate
28 g

Dietary Fiber 3 g

Sugars 22 g

Protein 1 g

French Toast Bites

Preparation Time:
5 minutes

Serves 2

Serving Size:
1 piece

Serve these kid-sized French toast squares for breakfast or a snack. Top them with mashed banana, crushed pineapple, a little Pear or Apple Spread (pp. 157 and 158), some low-fat vanilla yogurt, or some sugar-free pancake syrup.

2 slices whole-wheat or cracked wheat bread
1/4 cup liquid egg substitute
3 Tbsp low-fat (1%) milk
1/4 tsp vanilla extract
Pinch cinnamon or nutmeg
Pinch salt (optional)
Nonstick cooking spray

1. Cut each bread slice into 4 squares or triangles. In a medium shallow bowl or flat casserole, stir together the egg substitute, milk, vanilla, cinnamon, and salt (if desired).

2. Add the bread. With a large flat spoon or narrow blade spatula, gently move the squares around slightly to help them absorb the liquid. When about half the liquid has been absorbed, turn them and repeat the process until most of the egg mixture is used up.

3. Transfer the squares to a large nonstick spray-coated nonstick skillet preheated over medium heat. Brown each slice for 3 to 4 minutes, turning each over once with a narrow blade spatula during cooking. Serve plain or with a desired topping.

Exchanges
1 Starch

Calories 96
Calories from Fat 13
Total Fat 1 g
Saturated Fat 0 g
Cholesterol 1 mg
Sodium 214 mg
Total Carbohydrate 15 g
Dietary Fiber 2 g
Sugars 2 g
Protein 7 g

Holiday Wreaths

Preparation Time:
15 minutes

Serves 2

Serving Size:
1/2 bagel

Here's a fun way to observe the holiday season—with wreaths made from a bagel. It's surprising how much these edible wreaths look like the real thing. The recipe calls for dried chopped cranberries. If you like, you can use part cranberries and part chopped dried apricot for a multicolored effect.

1 whole-wheat or plain bagel cut in half and toasted, if desired
2 Tbsp fat-free cream cheese
3 Tbsp finely chopped fresh parsley leaves
1 tsp dried cranberries, chopped

1. Lay each bagel half on a plate. Spread each with half the cream cheese.

2. Sprinkle the parsley evenly over the cream cheese and press into place. Attractively arrange chopped cranberries on the surface of the wreaths.

Exchanges

2 Starch

Calories 179

Calories from Fat 9

Total Fat 1 g

Saturated Fat 0.1 g

Cholesterol 2 mg

Sodium 421 mg

Total Carbohydrate 33 g

Dietary Fiber 2 g

Sugars 2 g

Protein 8 g

Bread Puzzle

Preparation Time:
7 minutes

Serves 1

Here's the perfect snack for kids who like to play with their food—a bread slice puzzle! (Hint: To make it easy to spread refrigerated peanut butter, scoop it out of the jar with a plastic measuring spoon. Then lay the spoon in a microwave oven and microwave on high power for 5 to 10 seconds.)

1 slice whole-wheat bread, toasted

1/2 Tbsp peanut butter

1 Tbsp homemade Apple Spread (p. 158) or mashed banana or crushed juice-packed pineapple

1. Lay the toast slice on a cutting board. With a small, sharp knife, cut the bread into 2, 3, or 4 sections with tabs sticking from one section into the other, so that the pieces form a puzzle. Or cut a stair-step effect down the center of the bread slice. (It's easier to cut straight lines than curves.) Carefully separate the pieces to make sure they come apart.

2. Lay the puzzle pieces back in the original bread slice shape. Spread the sections with peanut butter and other desired topping. Mix up puzzle pieces and fit them back together before eating.

Exchanges

1 1/2 Starch

1/2 Fat

Calories 137

Calories from Fat 48

Total Fat 5 g

Saturated Fat 1 g

Cholesterol 0 mg

Sodium 185 mg

Total Carbohydrate 20 g

Dietary Fiber 3 g

Sugars 7 g

Protein 5 g

Serves 2

Serving Size:
1 slice

At the Zoo

Make snack time fun with an edible zoo, using toasted bread and cookie cutters. Or try other shapes for various holidays: hearts for Valentine's Day; stars, trees, and bells for the winter holidays; and shamrocks for St. Patrick's Day.

2–3 slices whole-wheat bread, toasted

1 Tbsp peanut butter or Neufchâtel cheese

1 Tbsp homemade Pear or Apple Spread (pp. 157 and 158) or 2 Tbsp mashed banana or 2 Tbsp crushed juice-packed pineapple

Raisins, currants, or dried apricots (optional)

Exchanges

1 Starch

1/2 Fat

Calories 107

Calories from Fat 45

Total Fat 5 g

Saturated Fat 1 g

Cholesterol 0 mg

Sodium 148 mg

Total Carbohydrate 13 g

Dietary Fiber 2 g

Sugars 3 g

Protein 4 g

1. Press the cookie cutters firmly into the toasted bread to make an animal or other shape. Spread with one or two of the suggested toppings. For even more fun, use raisins or currants for eyes and noses and a sliver of dried apricot for a mouth.

2. If you're making shamrocks, you can spread clover shapes with Neufchâtel and cover with finely chopped parsley leaves. You can use the same technique for a holiday tree and decorate it with raisins, dried cranberries, and chopped dried fruit. For hearts, mix a little red food coloring and a dash of cinnamon into Neufchâtel.

Hawaiian Pizza

Preparation Time:
5 minutes

Serves 2

Serving Size:
1 piece

Here's a fun "pizza" made with fruit instead of tomato sauce and cheese.

1 whole-wheat or oat bran English muffin or 2
  small whole-wheat pita bread rounds
1/4 cup fat-free vanilla yogurt
1/3 cup sliced fresh strawberries
3 Tbsp juice-packed crushed pineapple, well-
  drained

1. Toast the muffin halves. Spread with the yogurt.

2. Spoon the strawberries on the muffin halves.
   Sprinkle with the crushed pineapple.

Exchanges

1 Starch

1/2 Fruit

Calories 95

Calories from Fat 8

Total Fat 1 g

Saturated Fat 0 g

Cholesterol 1 mg

Sodium 128 mg

Total Carbohydrate
  19 g

Dietary Fiber 2 g

Sugars 7 g

Protein 4 g

Preparation Time:
3 minutes

Serves 2

Serving Size:
1 piece

Aladdin's Pizza

Aladdin would have loved these easy fruit and yogurt pizzas, which can also be made on toasted whole-wheat English muffin halves.

2 small pita bread rounds

1/4 cup reduced-fat vanilla yogurt

2 Tbsp chopped dried fruit, such as apricots, raisins, apples, or pears

1. Spread the pita bread rounds with yogurt.

2. Sprinkle with fruit. Serve immediately.

Exchanges

1 Starch

1 Fruit

Calories 145

Calories from Fat 8

Total Fat 1 g

Saturated Fat 0 g

Cholesterol 3 mg

Sodium 179 mg

Total Carbohydrate 31 g

Dietary Fiber 2 g

Sugars 12 g

Protein 4 g

Cinnamon Triangles

Preparation Time:
6 minutes

Serves 6

Serving Size:
5 triangles

Fun and easy to fix, these crispy treats are made with purchased wonton wrappers.

Nonstick cooking spray

2 tsp sugar

1/8 tsp cinnamon

15 wonton wrappers

1 1/2 tsp reduced-fat tub-style margarine
(4.5 g fat/T)

1. Preheat the oven to 400 degrees. Spray a small baking sheet with nonstick cooking spray. Set aside.

2. In a custard cup, mix together the sugar and cinnamon. Cut 15 wonton wrappers in half to form triangles and lay them on the baking sheet.

3. With your finger or the back of a spoon, brush the top of each wrapper with margarine, dividing it evenly. Sprinkle the cinnamon-sugar mixture over the top of each wrapper, dividing evenly.

4. Bake in the center of the oven for 3 to 4 minutes or until golden. Cool slightly before serving. Leftovers can be wrapped tightly and kept at room temperature for up to a week.

Exchanges
1/2 Starch

Calories 51
Calories from Fat 6
Total Fat 1 g
Saturated Fat 0 g
Cholesterol 3 mg
Sodium 93 mg
Total Carbohydrate 10 g
Dietary Fiber 1 g
Sugars 2 g
Protein 2 g

Preparation Time:
8 minutes

Serves 8

Serving Size:
1 turnover

Over-Easy Apple-Raisin Turnovers

1 1/2 tsp sugar

1/8 tsp cinnamon

1 medium apple, peeled or unpeeled, cored and cut into small cubes

1 Tbsp dark raisins

8 very fresh, reduced-calorie, whole-wheat bread slices

1. In a custard cup or on a small sheet of wax paper, stir together the sugar and cinnamon. In a 2-cup measure or similar small microwave-safe bowl, combine the sugar-cinnamon mixture, apple, and raisins. Stir to mix well.

2. Cover with wax paper and microwave on high power for 1 minute. Stir. Re-cover and microwave on high power for an additional 1 to 1 1/2 minutes or until the apples are softened. Meanwhile, trim the crusts from the bread slices and discard them. With a rolling pin, flatten the slices to 1/8 inch thick.

3. Place a generous tablespoon of apple mixture on one side of each bread slice and spread it out slightly. To form turnovers, fold the bread over the filling to make a triangle shape. Seal the edges by pressing with fork tines.

4. Lightly toast the slices in the toaster oven. Or toast under the broiler, browning lightly on one side and then the other. Cool slightly before eating. You can make up a batch of filling, use some of it immediately, and save the rest in the refrigerator. Then make additional turnovers over the next 2 to 3 days.

Exchanges

1/2 Carbohydrate

Calories 47

Calories from Fat 2

Total Fat 0 g

Saturated Fat 0 g

Cholesterol 0 mg

Sodium 75 mg

Total Carbohydrate 11 g

Dietary Fiber 2 g

Sugars 5 g

Protein 2 g

Banana Pops

Serves 6

Serving Size:
1 pop

Frozen banana pops are a snap to make and taste a lot like ice cream. For extra pizzazz, drizzle them with chocolate syrup before serving. The recipe calls for using popsicle sticks. If they are unavailable, the end of each pop can be held in a folded piece of plastic wrap.

6 small ripe bananas

6 popsicle sticks

6 Tbsp chocolate syrup (optional)

1. For each pop, carefully insert a popsicle stick into the bottom of 1 banana, burying about half of the stick. Wrap each banana individually in plastic wrap, and freeze for at least 6 hours.

2. To serve, unwrap each banana and eat like a popsicle. If desired, lay each banana on a plate and drizzle with 1 Tbsp of chocolate syrup before serving. To combat dripping chocolate, hold the pop over the plate while eating it.

3. Frozen banana pops will keep in the freezer, tightly wrapped, for 2 to 3 weeks.

Exchanges

1 Fruit

Calories 66

Calories from Fat 3

Total Fat 0 g

Saturated Fat 0 g

Cholesterol 0 mg

Sodium 1 mg

Total Carbohydrate 17 g

Dietary Fiber 2 g

Sugars 11 g

Protein 1 g

Microwave Wonders

For years I thought I didn't need a microwave. Then I finally got one and realized how useful it was for getting hot food on the table in a hurry. The recipes in this chapter, like Apple Spread, Sweet Potatoes Supreme, and Tangy Mustard Sauce, are designed exclusively for the microwave. In addition, there are others in the book, like the Apple Crisp, that use the microwave for part of the cooking process.

The recipes were all designed in my microwave, which is a high-powered model (900 watts) with a turntable. If your unit has less (or more) power, you may have to adjust the micro-waving time slightly. Also, if you do not have a turntable, stop and turn the container at least once during microwaving.

Remember that casserole and bowl sizes will make a difference in microwave cooking time. If you use a larger dish than the one specified, you may also have to cook the food longer. I often use a glass measuring cup for microwave cooking because I like the convenience of the handle. Although some people use plastic wrap to cover food being microwaved, I prefer wax paper, since I'm less likely to get burned by escaping steam. When plastic wrap comes in contact with microwaved food, molecules of plastic may be left on the surface of the food.

Homemade Pear Spread

Preparation Time:
7 minutes

Serves 16

Serving Size:
1 Tbsp

With a microwave and a food processor fitted with a circular shredder blade, you can make this tasty spread in a snap. Because it's very low in sugar, it makes a great substitute for jam or jelly. Be sure to cook only until the pears are softened and not runny.

1 1/2 cups (about 2 medium) grated or
    shredded, peeled fresh pear

2 tsp sugar

Scant 1/4 tsp ginger

1/2 tsp vanilla extract

1. In a 2-cup measure or similar small microwave-safe bowl, combine the pear, sugar, and ginger. Stir to mix well.

2. Cover with wax paper and microwave on high power for 2 minutes. Stir. Uncover and microwave for an additional 1 to 2 minutes on high power or until the pears are just soft. Stir in vanilla.

3. Serve warm or cover and refrigerate. The spread will keep in the refrigerator for 2 weeks.

Exchanges
Free

Calories 13

Calories from Fat 1

Total Fat 0 g

Saturated Fat 0 g

Cholesterol 0 mg

Sodium 0 mg

Total Carbohydrate
  3 g

Dietary Fiber 0 g

Sugars 3 g

Protein 0 g

Preparation Time:
10 minutes

Serves 16

Serving Size:
1 Tbsp

Homemade Apple Spread

Here's an easy apple spread I use as a topping for bagels or toast. It's mostly fruit, which makes it healthier than jam or even naturally sweetened commercial spreads. I make it with unpeeled apples, but you could peel them if you prefer.

2 cups (about 2 medium) grated or shredded sweet apples

2 Tbsp water

1 Tbsp sugar

1/4 tsp cinnamon

1. After shredding the apples, remove any large pieces of peel. In a 4-cup measure or similar medium microwave-safe bowl, combine the apples, water, sugar, and cinnamon. Stir to mix well.

2. Cover with wax paper and microwave on high power for 2 minutes. Stir. Re-cover and microwave for an additional 2 minutes. Stir, re-cover, and microwave for an additional minute, or until the apples are very soft and most of the water has been absorbed.

3. Serve warm, or cover and refrigerate. The spread will keep in the refrigerator for up to 2 weeks.

Exchanges

Free

Calories 13

Calories from Fat 1

Total Fat 0 g

Saturated Fat 0 g

Cholesterol 0 mg

Sodium 0 mg

Total Carbohydrate 3 g

Dietary Fiber 0 g

Sugars 3 g

Protein 0 g

Tangy Mustard Sauce

Preparation Time:
6 minutes

Serves 8

Serving Size:
1 Tbsp

This flavorful sauce tastes great as a sandwich spread in place of mayonnaise and mustard, mixed with turkey breast meat for a quick turkey salad, or on cooked vegetables, such as cauliflower or carrots.

1 Tbsp packed brown sugar

1 tsp dry mustard

1 Tbsp cider vinegar

1 Tbsp hot water

1/4 cup fat-free sour cream

2 Tbsp reduced-fat mayonnaise

1. In a small microwave-safe bowl, combine the sugar and mustard. Stir to mix well. Stir in the vinegar and water. Cover with wax paper and microwave on high power for 1 minute, or until the flavors are well blended.

2. Stir and cool slightly. Whisk in the sour cream and mayonnaise. Serve immediately, or cover and refrigerate for several hours before serving. The sauce will keep in the refrigerator for 4 to 5 days. Stir before serving.

Exchanges
1 Fat

Calories 26
Calories from Fat 10
Total Fat 1 g
Saturated Fat 0 g
Cholesterol 2 mg
Sodium 38 mg
Total Carbohydrate
3 g
Dietary Fiber 0 g
Sugars 3 g
Protein 1 g

Sweet Potatoes Supreme

Sweet potatoes make a great snack. They're high in beta-carotene and fiber. And they microwave beautifully —which means you can fix them in a jiffy.

1 medium sweet potato

2 Tbsp orange or pineapple juice

1/8 tsp ginger

2 Tbsp raisins or other dried fruit bits

2 tsp reduced-fat margarine

Exchanges

1 1/2 Starch

1/2 Fruit

Calories 138

Calories from Fat 15

Total Fat 2 g

Saturated Fat 0 g

Cholesterol 0 mg

Sodium 40 mg

Total Carbohydrate
30 g

Dietary Fiber 3 g

Sugars 17 g

Protein 2 g

1. Pierce the sweet potato with a fork and microwave on high power for 6 to 7 minutes or until tender. Meanwhile, in a 1-cup measure or similar small microwave-safe bowl, stir together the juice and ginger until well mixed. Stir in the raisins.

2. When the sweet potato is tender, remove it from the microwave. Then cover the juice mixture with wax paper and microwave it for 45 seconds to 1 minute on high power, or until heated through.

3. Meanwhile, cut the sweet potato in half and place on two plates. Mash the margarine into the flesh of each half with a fork. Pour the juice mixture over the sweet potato halves, mashing it into the flesh. Serve immediately.

Con Queso Bean Dip

Preparation Time:
10 minutes

Serves 20

Serving Size:
2 Tbsp

Keep this piquant Tex-Mex-style dip warm on a hot plate or return it to the microwave briefly to rewarm it.

1 15 1/2-oz can low-sodium or regular light red kidney beans, rinsed and well drained

3/4 cup mild or medium salsa

1 tsp chili powder

1 tsp cumin

1/8 tsp salt, or to taste (optional)

1 cup shredded reduced-fat Cheddar cheese

1/2 cup fat-free sour cream

2 Tbsp chopped chives or green onions

1. In a 1-quart microwave-safe casserole, mash the beans with a fork. Stir in the salsa, chili powder, cumin, and salt (if desired). Stir to mix well. Stir in the cheese.

2. Cover with the casserole lid and microwave on high power for 3 to 4 minutes until heated through. Remove from microwave. Stir to mix in the melted cheese. Spread the sour cream on top. Sprinkle with the chives.

3. Serve warm with fat-free tortilla chips. Cover and refrigerate leftovers, which will keep for 3 to 4 days.

Exchanges
1/2 Starch

Calories 44
Calories from Fat 12
Total Fat 1 g
Saturated Fat 1 g
Cholesterol 4 mg
Sodium 86 mg
Total Carbohydrate 5 g
Dietary Fiber 1 g
Sugars 1 g
Protein 3 g

Stuffing Pronto

Stuffing for a snack? Sure—if you love it as much as I do. This version, which features a variety of chopped vegetables, is so quick I can indulge myself any time I like. Check package labels to find a stuffing mix that's low in fat and salt.

1 small onion, chopped

1 large celery stalk, diced

1 cup diced cauliflower florets

5 or 6 baby carrots, thinly sliced

1/2 cup fat-free, low-sodium or regular chicken broth

2 Tbsp reduced-fat margarine

1/2 tsp poultry seasoning

Scant 1/4 tsp salt, or to taste (optional)

Dash black pepper

2 cups seasoned commercial crumb-style stuffing

Exchanges

1 Starch

1 Vegetable

Calories 109

Calories from Fat 15

Total Fat 2 g

Saturated Fat 0 g

Cholesterol 0 mg

Sodium 372 mg

Total Carbohydrate 19 g

Dietary Fiber 3 g

Sugars 3 g

Protein 3 g

1. In a medium microwave-safe bowl, combine all ingredients except the stuffing and stir to mix well. Cover with wax paper and microwave on high power for 4 to 5 minutes until the vegetables are tender, stopping and stirring the vegetables once during microwaving.

2. Remove the bowl from the microwave and stir in the stuffing mix until well combined. Cover and microwave for an additional 2 minutes on high power, stirring once. Serve warm. Leftovers can be stored in the refrigerator for 3 to 4 days.

Fruit Stuffing Pronto

Preparation Time:
9 minutes

Serves 6

Serving Size:
1/2 cup

Here's a quick and tasty variation on the stuffing theme, with apples and cranberries as well as vegetables.

1 small onion, chopped

1 medium celery stalk, diced

1 medium apple, cored and chopped

1/2 cup dried cranberries or raisins (or a mixture of the two)

1/2 cup fat-free, low-sodium or regular chicken broth

2 Tbsp reduced-fat margarine

Scant 1/4 tsp salt, or to taste (optional)

Dash black pepper

1/2 tsp poultry seasoning

2 cups seasoned commercial crumb-style stuffing

1. In a medium microwave-safe bowl, combine the onion, celery, apple, cranberries, broth, margarine, salt (if desired), and pepper. Stir to mix well. Cover with wax paper and microwave on high power for 4 to 5 minutes until the onion is tender, stopping and stirring the mixture once during microwaving.

2. Remove the bowl from the microwave and stir in the poultry seasoning. Then stir in the stuffing mix until well combined. Cover and microwave for an additional 2 minutes on high power, stopping and stirring once during microwaving.

3. Leftover stuffing will keep in the refrigerator for 2 to 3 days.

Exchanges

1 Starch

1 Fruit

Calories 145

Calories from Fat 15

Total Fat 2 g

Saturated Fat 0 g

Cholesterol 0 mg

Sodium 356 mg

Total Carbohydrate 28 g

Dietary Fiber 3 g

Sugars 12 g

Protein 3 g

Apple Scone Cake

Apples add flavor and texture to this quick and easy snack cake.

Nonstick cooking spray

3 Tbsp reduced-fat tub-style margarine (4.5 g fat/T)

1 tsp vanilla extract

3 Tbsp sugar

2 large egg whites

3/4 cup all-purpose white flour

1/4 cup oat bran

1 tsp baking powder

1/4 tsp cinnamon

1/8 tsp salt (optional)

1/4 cup low-fat buttermilk

1 large apple, cored, peeled, and thinly sliced

1 1/2 Tbsp sugar

1/4 tsp cinnamon

Exchanges

1 1/2 Carbohydrate

Calories 117

Calories from Fat 19

Total Fat 2 g

Saturated Fat 0 g

Cholesterol 0 mg

Sodium 101 mg

Total Carbohydrate 22 g

Dietary Fiber 1 g

Sugars 11 g

Protein 3 g

1. Spray an 8-inch round and at least 2-inch deep (or similar) microwave-safe glass dish with nonstick cooking spray. Set aside. In a large mixing bowl with an electric mixer on medium speed, beat together the margarine, vanilla, and sugar. Beat in the egg whites.

2. In a separate medium bowl, stir together the flour, oat bran, baking powder, cinnamon, and salt (if desired). Add the flour mixture and the buttermilk to the margarine mixture, beating until blended. Stir the apple into the batter.

3. Pour the batter into the prepared dish. Rap the dish against the countertop to remove any large air bubbles. Cover with wax paper and micro-wave on 70 percent power for 5 1/2 to 7 1/2 minutes, or until the cake top is just slightly soft when lightly pressed.

4. Mix together the sugar and cinnamon and sprinkle the mixture over the cake. Replace the wax paper and microwave for 1 to 1 1/2 minutes on high power until the sugar has melted and the cake springs back when pressed. Let stand for 5 minutes before serving.

Exchanges

1 1/2 Carbohydrate

1/2 Fat

Calories 128

Calories from Fat 32

Total Fat 4 g

Saturated Fat 0 g

Cholesterol 0 mg

Sodium 102 mg

Total Carbohydrate
21 g

Dietary Fiber 1 g

Sugars 10 g

Protein 3 g

Honey-Almond Scone Cake

Quick, easy, and full of flavor, this microwave dessert gets extra fiber from oat bran.

Nonstick cooking spray

3 Tbsp reduced-fat tub-style margarine
    (4.5 g fat/T)

1 tsp almond extract

3 Tbsp sugar

2 large egg whites

3/4 cup all-purpose white flour

1/4 cup oat bran

1 tsp baking powder

1/8 tsp salt (optional)

1/4 cup low-fat buttermilk

2 Tbsp mild or strong-flavored honey

1/4 tsp almond extract

3 Tbsp unblanched sliced almonds

1. Spray an 8-inch round and at least 2-inch deep (or similar) microwave-safe glass dish with non-stick cooking spray. Set aside. In a large mixing bowl with an electric mixer on medium speed, beat together the margarine, almond extract, and sugar. Beat in the egg whites.

2. In a separate medium bowl, stir together the flour, oat bran, baking powder, and salt (if desired). Add the flour mixture and the buttermilk to the margarine mixture, beating until blended.

3. Pour the batter into the prepared dish. Cover with wax paper and microwave on 70 percent power for 6 to 8 minutes, or until the cake top springs back when lightly pressed and a toothpick inserted in the center comes out clean. Remove the cake to a wire rack.

4. Mix together the honey and almond extract. With the back of a spoon, spread the mixture over the top of the warm cake. Sprinkle with the almonds. Let stand for 5 minutes before serving.

Serves 6

Serving Size:
1/2 cup

Apple Betty

*This is one of my favorite old recipes—updated and
made a lot healthier. If you want to use very fresh
bread, cut slices into cubes and let them dry out on the
cutting board for 30 to 40 minutes before using them.*

4 cups peeled, diced Red Delicious apples

3 cups 1/4- to 1/2-inch whole-wheat bread
    cubes

2 Tbsp packed brown sugar

2 Tbsp reduced-fat tub-style margarine
    (4.5 g fat/T)

1/2 tsp cinnamon

2 Tbsp hot water

Exchanges

1 1/2 Carbohydrate

1/2 Fat

Calories 119

Calories from Fat 22

Total Fat 2 g

Saturated Fat 0 g

Cholesterol 0 mg

Sodium 106 mg

Total Carbohydrate
25 g

Dietary Fiber 3 g

Sugars 17 g

Protein 2 g

1. Spread half the apples and bread cubes in the
   bottom of a nonstick 2-quart or similar microwave-
   safe casserole. Sprinkle with half the brown sugar.
   Dot with half of the margarine and sprinkle with
   half of the cinnamon.

2. Repeat with the remaining apples, bread cubes,
   brown sugar, margarine, and cinnamon. Stir to
   distribute the ingredients evenly. Sprinkle the
   water evenly over the top.

3. Cover the casserole with wax paper. Microwave
   on high power for 6 to 7 minutes. Uncover and
   stir. Microwave uncovered on high power for an
   additional 2 to 3 minutes, or until the apples are
   cooked through. The top will not be browned.

4. Serve warm. Top with a small dollop of fat-free
   yogurt or ice milk, if desired. Leftovers will
   keep, covered, at room temperature, for 2 days.

Delectable Desserts

Many people think there's no room for sweets in a healthy diet. But as researchers have learned more about the chemistry of food, they have come to the conclusion that sugars are not a special class of foods. They are just carbohydrates, and they are no more harmful than any other carbohydrates, such as potatoes, pasta, and bread.

This means that as long as you don't go overboard on sweets, you can include some sugar-containing foods in your healthy eating plan. When you do eat sugar-sweetened foods, you might try limiting the number of other carbohydrate foods you'll also be eating. For example, if you want to eat a serving of Apple Crisp or the Pumpkin Spice Muffins in this chapter, have them instead of a bread roll or a portion of pasta.

Not only have I kept sugar to a minimum in these recipes, I've also cut the fat and calories, so you can enjoy a serving of these treats without guilt. And I've taken advantage of the natural sugars in fruits, which are high in the vitamins, minerals, and fiber that should be included in your diet every day.

While many of the recipes in this chapter are made from scratch, some do take advantage of convenience foods available in your grocery store. Several, like the Apricot Kuchen and Pecan Buns, use refrigerator buttermilk biscuits. And you'll find elegant Pastry Cups and Cherry Tarts made from phyllo dough, which you can purchase in the frozen food section of most supermarkets.

By the way, you will find additional sweet treats in two other chapters: Just for Kids and Microwave Wonders.

Vanilla Custard

This wonderfully creamy custard tastes great by itself or with fruit. It's also used in the Cherry Tarts on page 173.

1/4 cup liquid egg substitute
1 cup low-fat (1%) milk
3/4 cup fat-free half-and-half
3 Tbsp sugar
2 Tbsp cornstarch
1 tsp regular margarine or butter
3/4 tsp vanilla extract

1. In a 2-cup glass measure or similar microwave-safe bowl, stir together the egg substitute, milk, and fat-free half-and-half with a fork. Cover with wax paper and microwave on high power for 2 to 2 1/2 minutes, stopping and stirring three times, until the mixture is hot but not boiling.

2. In the top of a double boiler, mix together the sugar and cornstarch. Place two or three inches of water in the bottom of the double boiler and heat over medium-high heat.

3. Place the top of the double boiler over the bottom. Adjust the heat so that the water in the bottom continues to boil but does not shoot out as steam. Gradually whisk the heated milk mixture into the sugar mixture, stirring vigorously until smooth. Cook over boiling water, stirring vigorously, for 3 to 4 minutes, or until the mixture thickens.

4. Remove from heat. Stir in the margarine and vanilla. Cool slightly. Serve warm, or cover and refrigerate for 3 to 4 hours or up to 48 hours.

Exchanges

1 Carbohydrate

1/2 Fat

Calories 99

Calories from Fat 15

Total Fat 2 g

Saturated Fat 0.7 g

Cholesterol 5 mg

Sodium 92 mg

Total Carbohydrate
  16 g

Dietary Fiber 0 g

Sugars 12 g

Protein 4 g

Pastry Cups

Preparation Time:
15 minutes

Serves 12

Serving Size:
1 cup

Virtually fat-free, these elegant but easy phyllo cups make the perfect shell for a variety of desserts. Fill them with cut fruit or make the rich-tasting Cherry Tarts on page 173.

Butter-flavored nonstick cooking spray
3 large phyllo sheets, thawed

1. Spray a 12-cup standard muffin tin with butter-flavored nonstick cooking spray. Set aside. Preheat the oven to 400 degrees.

2. Lay the phyllo on a large plastic cutting board or other flat surface. Using sharp scissors or a sharp knife, cut each pastry sheet into 4- to 4 1/2-inch squares. Stack the squares and keep them covered with wax paper until you are ready for them.

3. Spray 3 squares with butter-flavored nonstick cooking spray. Place the squares on top of each other, rotating them slightly so that the corners are facing in different directions. Gently press the squares into a muffin cup, making a basket. Repeat the process to make 12 cups.

4. Bake on the center oven rack for 4 to 5 minutes or until the edges of the cups begin to crisp. Cups can be cooled slightly and filled with desired filling. Or they can be cooled, covered with plastic wrap, and stored in the refrigerator for 3 to 4 days before filling. They should not be filled until 2 to 3 hours before serving.

Exchanges
Free

Calories 18
Calories from Fat 1
Total Fat 0 g
Saturated Fat 0 g
Cholesterol 0 mg
Sodium 30 mg
Total Carbohydrate
4 g
Dietary Fiber 0 g
Sugars 0 g
Protein 1 g

Preparation Time:
10 minutes

Serves 6

Serving Size:
1 cup

Pear Cups

With phyllo dough, you can quickly make these easy and festive baked pear tarts.

Butter-flavored nonstick cooking spray
1 1/2 large phyllo sheets, thawed
6 juice-packed canned pear halves
2 tsp sugar
1/8 tsp cinnamon

1. Spray a 6-cup standard muffin tin with butter-flavored nonstick cooking spray. Preheat the oven to 400 degrees.

2. Lay the phyllo on a large plastic cutting board or other flat surface. Using sharp scissors or a sharp knife, cut each pastry sheet into six 4- to 4 1/2-inch squares. Keep the squares covered with wax paper until you are ready for them.

3. Spray 3 squares with butter-flavored nonstick cooking spray. Place the squares on top of each other, rotating them slightly so that the corners are facing in different directions. Gently press the squares into a muffin cup, making a basket. Repeat the process to make 6 cups.

4. Lay a pear half, cut side up, in each cup. Mix together the sugar and cinnamon. Sprinkle each pear lightly with the mixture, dividing evenly. Bake on the center oven rack for 5 to 6 minutes or until the edges of the cups begin to crisp. Cool slightly on a wire rack. Serve warm. Leftover cups can be covered and refrigerated for 3 to 4 days. They can be served chilled.

Exchanges

1 Fruit

Calories 54

Calories from Fat 1

Total Fat 0 g

Saturated Fat 0 g

Cholesterol 0 mg

Sodium 33 mg

Total Carbohydrate 13 g

Dietary Fiber 1 g

Sugars 7 g

Protein 1 g

Cherry Tarts

Preparation Time:
20 minutes

Serves 12

Serving Size:
1 tart

For an elegant end to a special meal—or a wonderful tea-time treat—try this sumptuous cherry tart.

1 20-oz can lite cherry pie filling
1/4 tsp cinnamon
1 recipe pastry cups (p. 171)
1 recipe vanilla custard (p. 170)

1. Stir together the cherry pie filling and cinnamon. Set aside.

2. Set each pastry shell on a serving plate. Spoon 2 Tbsp of custard into each. Spoon 2 1/2 Tbsp of cherry pie filling over custard.

3. Serve at once. Or fill shells up to 2 hours before needed and refrigerate.

Exchanges
1 Carbohydrate

Calories 91
Calories from Fat 12
Total Fat 1 g
Saturated Fat 1 g
Cholesterol 20 mg
Sodium 60 mg
Total Carbohydrate 18 g
Dietary Fiber 1 g
Sugars 12 g
Protein 2 g

Preparation Time:
20 minutes

Serves 8

Serving Size:
1 piece

Here's a wonderful late summer combination—peaches with a biscuit topping. Starting the fruit in the microwave gives the peaches a well-baked taste and texture.

3 Tbsp sugar

2 Tbsp white flour

1/4 tsp cinnamon

4 cups peeled and sliced ripe peaches

1 cup white flour

1 Tbsp sugar

1 1/2 tsp baking powder

1/8 tsp salt

3 Tbsp reduced-fat margarine

1/2 cup low-fat (1%) milk

1. Preheat the oven to 400 degrees. In a microwave-safe, oven-proof 2-quart casserole, combine the sugar, flour, and cinnamon. Add the peaches and stir until all of the flour mixture coats the peaches. Cover with the casserole lid and microwave on high power for about 4 minutes, stirring twice, or until the peaches have softened and are surrounded by a thickened sauce. Reserve the peaches in the microwave.

2. In a medium bowl, combine the flour, sugar, baking powder, and salt. Stir to mix well. With a fork or fingers, blend in margarine until completely incorporated. Stir in the milk. The batter will be slightly soupy.

Exchanges

2 Carbohydrate

Calories 140

Calories from Fat 18

Total Fat 2 g

Saturated Fat 0 g

Cholesterol 1 mg

Sodium 146 mg

Total Carbohydrate
28 g

Dietary Fiber 2 g

Sugars 13 g

Protein 3 g

3. Remove the casserole from the microwave. Divide the dough into 8 portions (about 2 Tbsp each). Drop the dough onto the hot peach mixture. Bake in the preheated oven for 18 to 25 minutes or until the filling is bubbly and the topping is set and beginning to brown. Cool for 5 minutes before serving.

4. The cobbler is best served warm. It will keep, covered, at room temperature for about 2 days.

Apricot Kuchen

Here's a delicious, practically instant apricot kuchen, with a crust made from refrigerator buttermilk biscuits. When measuring out the apricot preserves, use plastic measuring spoons so that they can go in the microwave.

Nonstick cooking spray

1 15-oz can juice-packed apricot halves

1 7 1/2-oz package reduced-fat refrigerator buttermilk biscuits

1 tsp reduced-fat tub-style margarine (4.5 g fat/T)

1 1/2 Tbsp apricot preserves

1 Tbsp sugar

1. Preheat the oven to 450 degrees. Spray a 9-inch pie plate with nonstick cooking spray. Set aside. Drain the apricots well in a colander. Blot them dry with paper towels.

2. Open the biscuit carton and separate the biscuits. Place them on the pie plate and press and squeeze the inner edges together so that they touch and cover the bottom of the plate. With your finger or the back of a spoon, spread the margarine on the biscuits, dividing it evenly.

3. Lay the measuring spoons of apricot preserves on a plate and microwave at full power for 10 to 15 seconds to soften. Drizzle the melted preserves over the margarine and spread it evenly with the back of the spoon.

Exchanges

1 1/2 Carbohydrate

Calories 98

Calories from Fat 10

Total Fat 1 g

Saturated Fat 0 g

Cholesterol 0 mg

Sodium 232 mg

Total Carbohydrate 21 g

Dietary Fiber 1 g

Sugars 9 g

Protein 2 g

4. Arrange the apricot halves, cut side down, in an attractive pattern over the biscuits. Sprinkle the kuchen top evenly with the sugar.

5. Bake in the center of the oven for 11 to 13 minutes or until the edges of the biscuits are well browned and the liquid at the edge of the plate is bubbly. Serve hot. Leftover kuchen will keep for 1 to 2 days at room temperature, if tightly wrapped.

Noodle Pudding

Preparation Time:
20 minutes

Serves 20

Serving Size:
1 piece

Serve this tasty pudding to a crowd of hungry snackers. The recipe uses flat, yolkless noodles.

Nonstick cooking spray

6 cups uncooked medium-sized reduced-fat egg noodles (about 7 1/2 oz)

6 oz Neufchâtel cream cheese, at room temperature

1/3 cup plus 2 Tbsp Splenda, divided

1 1/4 cups liquid egg substitute

1 cup fat-free ricotta cheese

1 Tbsp vanilla extract

1/4 tsp salt (optional)

1 cup shredded fat-free mozzarella cheese

1 8-oz can crushed juice-packed pineapple, well-drained

1/2 cup dried cranberries or raisins

1/4 tsp ground cinnamon

Exchanges

1 Carbohydrate

1/2 Fat

Calories 104

Calories from Fat 18

Total Fat 2 g

Saturated Fat 1.2 g

Cholesterol 11 mg

Sodium 148 mg

Total Carbohydrate 13 g

Dietary Fiber 1 g

Sugars 5 g

Protein 7 g

1. Preheat the oven to 375 degrees. Spray a 9- by 13-inch baking pan with nonstick cooking spray and set aside. Cook noodles according to package directions. Drain well.

2. Meanwhile, in a large mixer bowl, combine the Neufchâtel cream cheese and 1/3 cup Splenda. Beat on medium speed until well combined and smooth. Add the egg substitute, ricotta, vanilla, and salt, if desired. Beat on medium speed. When partially combined, increase speed to high and beat until well mixed.

3. Stir in the mozzarella, pineapple, and dried cranberries. Stir in the noodles. Turn out into the prepared dish and spread evenly, using the back of a large spoon. Stir together the additional Splenda and the cinnamon. Sprinkle the mixture evenly over the noodle mixture.

4. Bake for 33 to 38 minutes until just set and a toothpick inserted in the center comes out clean. Do not overbake.

Preparation Time:
20 minutes

Serves 12

Serving Size:
1 muffin

Cranberry-Orange Muffins

Here's a fruit muffin you can enjoy as a snack or for breakfast.

Nonstick cooking spray

1/4 cup dried cranberries

1/3 cup orange juice

1 1/3 cups all-purpose white flour

3/4 cup whole-wheat flour

1/3 cup sugar

2 1/2 tsp baking powder

1/8 tsp ginger

1/8 tsp salt

1 cup low-fat (1%) milk

1 large egg white

1/4 cup canola or safflower oil

2 tsp vanilla extract

Exchanges

1 1/2 Carbohydrate

1 Fat

Calories 162

Calories from Fat 47

Total Fat 5 g

Saturated Fat 0 g

Cholesterol 1 mg

Sodium 116 mg

Total Carbohydrate
26 g

Dietary Fiber 1 g

Sugars 9 g

Protein 4 g

1. Preheat the oven to 425 degrees. Coat a 12-cup standard muffin tin with nonstick cooking spray and set aside. Chop the cranberries. In a 2-cup microwave-safe measure, combine the cranberries and orange juice. Cover with wax paper and microwave on high power for 1 minute, or until the cranberries are softened. Set aside.

2. In a large bowl, stir together the white flour, whole-wheat flour, sugar, baking powder, ginger, and salt. Add the milk, egg white, oil, and vanilla to the measuring cup with the cranberry-orange mixture. Stir with a fork until well mixed.

3. Gently stir the cranberry mixture into the dry ingredients until just incorporated. Do not over-mix. Divide the batter evenly among the muffin cups. (They will be almost full.) Bake on the center oven rack for 15 to 18 minutes, or until the muffins are lightly browned and a toothpick inserted in the center of one comes out clean. Transfer the pan to a wire rack, and let it stand for 5 minutes before removing the muffins.

4. The muffins will keep for 1 to 2 days at room temperature if tightly wrapped. Freeze for longer storage.

Preparation Time:
20 minutes

Serves 12

Serving Size:
1 muffin

Pineapple-Carrot Muffins

I love the combination of tastes and textures in these muffins, which make a great snack or a quick breakfast. You can make them with clover honey, but they're more flavorful with a stronger-flavored honey, such as locust or buckwheat.

Nonstick cooking spray

1 cup all-purpose white flour

3/4 cup whole-wheat flour

3 Tbsp sugar

2 tsp baking powder

1/2 tsp baking soda

1 tsp cinnamon

1/8 tsp cloves

1/8 tsp salt (optional)

Scant 1 cup low-fat buttermilk

3 Tbsp canola or olive oil

1 large egg white

2 Tbsp mild or strong-flavored honey

1 8-oz can juice-packed crushed pineapple, well drained

1 medium carrot, grated or shredded

1/2 cup dark seedless raisins

1. Preheat the oven to 400 degrees. Coat a 12-cup standard muffin tin with nonstick cooking spray and set aside. In a medium bowl, combine the flours, sugar, baking powder, baking soda, cinnamon, cloves, and salt (if desired) and stir to mix well.

Exchanges

2 Carbohydrate

1/2 Fat

Calories 158

Calories from Fat 36

Total Fat 4 g

Saturated Fat 0 g

Cholesterol 1 mg

Sodium 146 mg

Total Carbohydrate
28 g

Dietary Fiber 2 g

Sugars 13 g

Protein 3 g

2. In a small bowl, blend the buttermilk, oil, egg white, and honey with a fork. Add to the dry mixture and stir to incorporate, but do not overmix. Stir in the pineapple, shredded carrot, and raisins. Divide the batter evenly among muffin tin cups. (Cups will be almost full.)

3. Bake for 22 to 25 minutes or until the tops of the muffins are browned. The muffins taste best warm and fresh but will keep for 1 to 2 days at room temperature if tightly wrapped. Freeze for longer storage.

Preparation Time:
15 minutes

Serves 12

Serving Size:
1 muffin

Pumpkin Spice Muffins

If you like gingerbread, you'll love these muffins!

Nonstick cooking spray

1 cup oat bran

1 cup all-purpose white flour

1/4 cup sugar

1 tsp baking powder

1/2 tsp baking soda

1 tsp pumpkin pie spice

1/8 tsp salt

1/4 cup liquid egg substitute

1/2 cup low-fat buttermilk

1/2 cup canned solid-pack pumpkin (not pumpkin pie filling)

3 Tbsp canola or corn oil

2 Tbsp dark molasses

3/4 cup dark or light raisins

Exchanges

2 Carbohydrate

1/2 Fat

Calories 159

Calories from Fat 39

Total Fat 4 g

Saturated Fat 0 g

Cholesterol 0 mg

Sodium 131 mg

Total Carbohydrate
27 g

Dietary Fiber 2 g

Sugars 13 g

Protein 4 g

1. Preheat the oven to 400 degrees. Coat a 12-cup standard muffin tin with nonstick cooking spray and set aside. In a large bowl, combine the oat bran, flour, sugar, baking powder, baking soda, pumpkin pie spice, and salt. Stir to mix well.

2. Add the egg substitute, buttermilk, pumpkin, oil, and molasses. Stir until just mixed. Stir in the raisins. Spoon the batter into the muffin tin cups. Bake for 16 to 19 minutes, or until the muffins are springy to the touch and lightly browned.

3. Cool for 2 to 3 minutes and remove. Serve warm or store at room temperature in an airtight container for 2 to 3 days. Freeze for longer storage.

Apple Crisp

Preparation Time:
18 minutes

Serves 8

Serving Size:
1/2 cup

If you like cooked apples, you'll love the taste of this easy crisp. Starting the apples in the microwave gives them a well-baked texture.

6 cups thinly sliced, peeled, tart apples

2 Tbsp all-purpose white flour

1 Tbsp sugar

1/2 tsp cinnamon

Nonstick cooking spray

1/2 cup quick-cooking rolled oats

1/4 cup all-purpose white flour

3 Tbsp packed light brown sugar

2 Tbsp reduced-fat tub-style margarine
(4.5 g fat/T)

1. Preheat the oven to 400 degrees. In a large bowl, combine the apples, 2 Tbsp flour, sugar, and cinnamon. Stir to mix well. Transfer the mixture to a nonstick spray–coated 10-inch microwave-safe pie plate. Cover with wax paper and microwave on high power for about 4 minutes or until the apples are partially cooked.

2. Meanwhile, for the topping, in a medium bowl, combine the oats, flour, and brown sugar. Mix well with a fork or fingers. Blend in margarine with a fork or fingers until completely incorporated. Distribute the topping over the apples.

3. Bake in the oven for 22 to 28 minutes or until the apples are tender when pierced with a fork and the filling is bubbly. Leftovers can be stored covered, at room temperature, for 2 to 3 days.

Exchanges

2 Carbohydrate

Calories 144

Calories from Fat 17

Total Fat 2 g

Saturated Fat 0 g

Cholesterol 0 mg

Sodium 25 mg

Total Carbohydrate
32 g

Dietary Fiber 3 g

Sugars 22 g

Protein 2 g

Blueberry Muffins

Preparation Time:
12 minutes

Serves 12

Serving Size:
1 muffin

These are packed with flavor and fiber!

Nonstick cooking spray
1 cup all-purpose white flour
1 cup oat bran
1/3 cup sugar
1 1/2 tsp baking powder
1/2 tsp baking soda
1/2 tsp lemon zest
1/8 tsp salt
3 Tbsp reduced-fat tub-style margarine (4.5 g fat/T)
1 large egg white
1 cup low-fat buttermilk
1/8 tsp lemon extract
1 1/4 cups fresh or dry-packed (unsweetened) frozen blueberries

Exchanges

1 1/2 Carbohydrate

Calories 115
Calories from Fat 18
Total Fat 2 g
Saturated Fat 0 g
Cholesterol 1 mg
Sodium 173 mg
Total Carbohydrate 21 g
Dietary Fiber 2 g
Sugars 8 g
Protein 4 g

1. Preheat the oven to 400 degrees. Spray a 12-cup standard muffin tin with nonstick cooking spray and set aside. In a large bowl, combine the flour, oat bran, sugar, baking powder, baking soda, lemon zest, and salt and stir to mix well.

2. With a pastry cutter or two forks, blend in the margarine until it is completely incorporated and the mixture resembles coarse meal. Add the egg white, buttermilk, and lemon extract. Stir until just mixed. Gently stir in the blueberries.

3. Divide batter evenly among the muffin cups. Bake for 16 to 20 minutes or until nicely browned. Remove to a wire rack. Serve warm. Muffins will keep at room temperature for 2 to 3 days if tightly wrapped.

Cinnamon Biscuits

Preparation Time:
6 minutes

Serves 6

Serving Size:
1 biscuit

A little sugar and margarine go a long way on these fun and easy-to-make cinnamon biscuits. Note that I've used a small package of biscuits for this very quick but very tasty recipe.

Nonstick cooking spray

1 1/2 tsp sugar

Generous pinch cinnamon

1 4 1/2-oz package reduced-fat refrigerator
 buttermilk biscuits

1 tsp reduced-fat tub-style margarine
 (4.5 g fat/T)

1. Preheat the oven to 450 degrees. Spray a small baking sheet with nonstick cooking spray and set aside.

2. In a custard cup, mix together the sugar and cinnamon. Open the biscuit carton and separate the biscuits. Set the biscuits on the baking sheet.

3. With your finger or the back of a spoon, brush the top of each biscuit with margarine, dividing it evenly. Sprinkle the cinnamon-sugar mixture over the top of each biscuit, dividing it evenly.

4. Bake in the center of the oven for 8 to 10 minutes or until golden. Serve hot.

Exchanges
1/2 Starch

Calories 56
Calories from Fat 9
Total Fat 1 g
Saturated Fat 0 g
Cholesterol 0 mg
Sodium 185 mg
Total Carbohydrate 11 g
Dietary Fiber 0 g
Sugars 2 g
Protein 1 g

Pecan Buns

Preparation Time:
4 minutes

Serves 10

Serving Size:
1 bun

You won't believe how easy it is to make these rich-tasting pecan buns. You can use mild honey, but one with a stronger taste, such as buckwheat, will add more flavor to the buns.

Nonstick cooking spray

1 7 1/2-oz package reduced-fat refrigerator buttermilk biscuits

1 tsp reduced-fat tub-style margarine (4.5 g fat/T)

1 1/2 Tbsp mild or strong-flavored honey

2 Tbsp finely chopped pecans

1. Preheat the oven to 450 degrees. Spray a 9-inch pie plate with nonstick cooking spray and set aside.

2. Open the biscuit carton and separate the biscuits. Place them on the pie plate so that they are barely touching.

3. With your finger or the back of a spoon, spread the margarine on the biscuits, dividing it evenly. Pour the honey on the biscuits, dividing it evenly, and spread it to cover the biscuit tops. Sprinkle the biscuits with the pecans.

4. Bake in the center of the oven for 8 to 10 minutes or until golden. Serve hot. Leftover buns will keep at room temperature for 1 to 2 days, if tightly covered. They can be served as is or rewarmed quickly in the microwave or toaster oven.

Exchanges

1 Carbohydrate

Calories 69

Calories from Fat 15

Total Fat 2 g

Saturated Fat 0 g

Cholesterol 0 mg

Sodium 183 mg

Total Carbohydrate 13 g

Dietary Fiber 0 g

Sugars 4 g

Protein 1 g

Apple-Cranberry Turnovers

Use refrigerator biscuits for a quick dessert!

Nonstick cooking spray

1 medium apple, peeled, cored, and diced

2 Tbsp dried cranberries

1 Tbsp sugar

1/4 tsp cinnamon

2 Tbsp water

1 7 1/2-oz package reduced-fat refrigerator buttermilk biscuits

1. Preheat the oven to 400 degrees. Spray a baking sheet with nonstick cooking spray and set aside.

2. In a 2-cup measure or similar small microwave-safe bowl, combine the apple, cranberries, sugar, and cinnamon. Stir to mix. Stir in the water. Cover with wax paper and microwave on high power for 3 minutes, stopping and stirring once during microwaving. Cool slightly.

3. Working on a nonstick spray–coated surface, flatten each biscuit into a three-inch round. Spoon about 2 tsp of the mixture into the center of the biscuit. Fold the biscuit in half over the filling, making a turnover shape. Seal the edges by pressing closed with fingers and then with the tines of a fork. Lay the biscuits on the prepared baking sheet. Prick the top of each turnover with the fork tines.

4. Bake for 8 to 10 minutes, or until the tops of the biscuits begin to brown. Serve hot. Leftovers will keep for 1 to 2 days, tightly covered, at room temperature.

Preparation Time: 10 minutes

Serves 10

Serving Size: 1 turnover

Exchanges

1 Carbohydrate

Calories 68

Calories from Fat 7

Total Fat 1 g

Saturated Fat 0 g

Cholesterol 0 mg

Sodium 180 mg

Total Carbohydrate 14 g

Dietary Fiber 1 g

Sugars 5 g

Protein 1 g

More Scrumptious Snacks

These recipes feature the use of monounsaturated and poly-unsaturated fats found in oils, such as canola oil and olive oil, and in nuts. Nuts add great flavor and excellent nutrition to many snacks. Enjoy some crisp Cabbage and Peanut Slaw. Or try the Summer Cheesecake with its crunchy pie crust made of ground pecans.

I like to serve mini-meals, so my snacks are especially hearty and good. These recipes are tasty enough to serve to your favorite guests and easy enough to make just for yourself. There are plenty of dips to offer at your next party and some delicious desserts, like Marzipan Candy and Red, White, and Blue Fruit Tart.

Red, White, and Green Bean Dip

Beans are a wonderful food, high in flavor and fiber. Serve this dip with whole-wheat pita bread triangles or whole-wheat crackers.

1 19-oz can cannellini beans, rinsed and drained

2 1/2 Tbsp extra-virgin olive oil

2 Tbsp chopped parsley leaves

2 Tbsp chopped chives or sliced green onions

1 Tbsp lemon juice

1/2 tsp dried rosemary leaves

1 tsp chopped garlic

1/4 tsp salt, or to taste (optional)

1/8 tsp white pepper

2 Tbsp chopped pimiento

1. In a food processor, combine the beans, oil, parsley, chives, lemon juice, rosemary, garlic, salt (if using), and pepper. Process until smooth. Stir in pimiento.

2. Serve at once or cover and refrigerate until chilled. Dip will keep in the refrigerator 2 to 3 days.

Preparation Time: 12 minutes

Serves 11

Serving Size: 2 Tbsp

Exchanges

1/2 Starch

1/2 Fat

Calories 73

Calories from Fat 29

Total Fat 3 g

Saturated Fat 0 g

Calories from Fat 29

Cholesterol 0 mg

Sodium 89 mg

Total Carbohydrate 8 g

Dietary Fiber 2 g

Sugars 0 g

Protein 3 g

Salsa Bean Dip

Serves 14

Serving Size:
  2 Tbsp

This easy Southwestern-style bean dip is high in taste appeal. To get the right texture, you must drain the salsa. The preparation time looks long, but much of this time includes draining the salsa. You can use either mild or medium salsa in the dip. If you use mild and find you'd like it spicier, add a bit of hot sauce.

3/4 cup mild or medium thick and chunky salsa

1 19-oz can cannellini beans, rinsed and
    drained

1 tsp lemon juice

1 tsp dark chili powder (or to taste)

1 tsp ground cumin

1/8 tsp salt

Exchanges

1/2 Starch

1. Place the salsa in a sieve over a large bowl. Tap the sieve occasionally to help the salsa drain until the chunky part remains in the sieve, about 3 to 4 minutes. Discard the liquid.

Calories 36

Calories from Fat 2

Total Fat 0 g

2. In the bowl, mash the beans slightly with a fork.

Saturated Fat 0 g

3. Add the chunky portion of the salsa, lemon juice, chili powder, cumin, and salt. Stir until combined. Transfer to a serving bowl.

Cholesterol 0 mg

Sodium 74 mg

Total Carbohydrate
  7 g

4. Serve at once or cover and refrigerate for several hours. Serve with baked corn chips. Leftover dip will keep in the refrigerator for 3 to 4 days.

Dietary Fiber 2 g

Sugars 0 g

Protein 2 g

Blue Cheese Spread

Preparation Time:
12 minutes

Serves 32

Serving Size:
2 tsp

Here's a cheese spread with crowd appeal. My guests love the mild blue cheese flavor and the crunch of pecans and celery.

5 oz reduced-fat cream cheese
3 oz fat-free cream cheese
1/2 cup crumbled blue cheese
1 tsp instant minced onion
Dash garlic powder
1 large stalk celery, finely diced
1/4 cup finely chopped pecans

1. In a medium bowl, combine the cream cheeses, blue cheese, onion, and garlic powder.

2. Mash and stir with a fork until mixed. Stir in the celery and pecans. Transfer to a serving bowl. Serve at once or cover with plastic wrap and refrigerate for 1 to 2 hours. Cheese spread will keep in the refrigerator for up to a week.

Exchanges

1/2 Fat

Calories 26

Calories from Fat 19

Total Fat 2 g

Saturated Fat 1 g

Cholesterol 5 mg

Sodium 59 mg

Total Carbohydrate
1 g

Dietary Fiber 0 g

Sugars 0 g

Protein 1 g

Antipasto

Preparation Time:
15 minutes

Serves 8

Serving Size:
3/4 cup

If you like Italian-style antipasto, try this easy version. It's perfect for a company appetizer. Or whip up a batch and keep it in the refrigerator, just for the family. I like the taste of freshly made dressing with this dish, but if you prefer, you can use low-fat bottled Italian dressing. Rather than using Italian cold cuts, which tend to be quite high in fat, I've substituted cooked lean Canadian bacon.

Dressing:

1/4 cup olive oil, preferably extra virgin

1/2 Tbsp water

2 tsp lemon juice

1 tsp red wine vinegar

1 tsp Italian seasoning

Vegetables and Meat:

1 14 1/2-oz can artichoke heart quarters, well drained

2 cups grape tomatoes

1 coarsely sliced celery stalk

1/2 red pepper, seeded and cut into strips

1/2 yellow pepper, seeded and cut into strips

3 oz cooked lean Canadian bacon, cut into thin strips

1. In a large bowl, combine the oil, water, lemon juice, vinegar, and Italian seasoning. Stir to mix well.

Exchanges

1 Vegetable

1 1/2 Fat

Calories 102

Calories from Fat 71

Total Fat 8 g

Saturated Fat 1 g

Cholesterol 5 mg

Sodium 233 mg

Total Carbohydrate 6 g

Dietary Fiber 1 g

Sugars 2 g

Protein 3 g

2. Remove any coarse outer leaves from the artichoke hearts. Stir the artichoke hearts, tomatoes, celery, peppers, and Canadian bacon into the dressing and gently toss to coat.

3. If desired, transfer to a shallow serving dish or platter. Serve at once, or cover and refrigerate for up to 24 hours. Antipasto will keep in the refrigerator for 3 to 4 days.

Cabbage and Peanut Slaw

I like cole slaw so much that I look for interesting ways to enliven the texture and flavor. You can add various vegetables to the mix, but I also love this one that features peanuts.

1/3 cup reduced-fat mayonnaise

1 1/2 Tbsp cider vinegar

1 1/2 Tbsp Splenda

5 cups very thinly sliced green cabbage

1/4 cup unsalted or salted peanuts, coarsely chopped

2 Tbsp chopped red onion

Exchanges

1 Vegetable

1 1/2 Fat

1. In a medium-large bowl, stir together the mayonnaise, vinegar, and Splenda.

2. Add the cabbage, peanuts, and onion. Stir to mix well. Serve immediately, or cover and refrigerate for up to 24 hours before serving. Cole slaw will keep in the refrigerator for 3 or 4 days.

Calories 99

Calories from Fat 70

Total Fat 8 g

Saturated Fat 1.2 g

Cholesterol 4 mg

Sodium 124 mg

Total Carbohydrate
6 g

Dietary Fiber 2 g

Sugars 3 g

Protein 3 g

Red, White, and Blue Fruit Tart

Preparation Time:
30 minutes

Serves 8

Serving Size:
1/8 tart

I love to serve this dessert for company, although I always hope there will be leftovers for me! I've made the crust of the tart from ground almonds. If you like marzipan, you'll love the taste. I like to use strawberries and blueberries for the topping. But you could substitute peaches or raspberries, if you like.

1 marzipan crust (see recipe, p. 205)
3 oz fat-free or reduced-fat cream cheese, at room temperature
1 Tbsp reduced-fat (2%) milk
1 Tbsp Splenda
1 cup washed, hulled, and sliced strawberries
1/2 cup blueberries, washed and picked over

1. Make marzipan crust. Set aside.

2. In a small bowl, combine the cream cheese, milk, and Splenda with a spoon. Stir until uniform and spread the mixture over the prepared crust.

3. Attractively arrange the fruit over the cream cheese mixture. For example, make a circle of blueberries around the outside and mound the additional berries in the center. Then add two rings of sliced strawberries in the remaining space. Refrigerate.

4. When cool, cover with plastic wrap, or serve immediately. The tart can be made up to 12 hours before serving. It will keep in the refrigerator for 2 to 3 days, but the cream cheese layer may start to absorb color from the fruit after 24 hours. Alternatively, you can make the crust the day before and then complete the tart before serving.

Exchanges
1/2 Carbohydrate
1 Very Lean Meat
2 Fat

Calories 160
Calories from Fat 103
Total Fat 11 g
Saturated Fat 0.9 g
Cholesterol 1 mg
Sodium 89 mg
Total Carbohydrate 9 g
Dietary Fiber 3 g
Sugars 4 g
Protein 7 g

Serves 6

Serving Size:
1/6 tart

Cranberry-Orange Tart

*Fresh cranberries give this tart its wonderful tang.
Since they are only available in the fall, I buy a lot of
them and freeze them for later use. To speed the jelling
of the cranberry mixture, you can put the saucepan in
the freezer, but check it periodically to make sure the
mixture doesn't freeze. The marzipan crust tastes
wonderful with the cranberries.*

1 marzipan crust (see recipe, p. 205)

1 1/3 cups fresh cranberries, washed and
picked over

1 cup Splenda

1 cup hot water, divided

1 packet unflavored gelatin

1 tsp vanilla extract

1/2 tsp orange extract

Exchanges

3 Fat

1 Carbohydrate

Calories 212

Calories from Fat
132

Total Fat 15 g

Saturated Fat 0 g

Cholesterol 0 mg

Sodium 25 mg

Total Carbohydrate
15 g

Dietary Fiber 5 g

Sugars 8 g

Protein 7 g

1. Make marzipan crust. Set aside.

2. In a food processor, chop the cranberries until
finely chopped.

3. Transfer the cranberries to a medium saucepan.
Stir in the Splenda and 1/2 cup of the water.
Bring to a boil. Reduce the heat and simmer,
uncovered, for 10 to 15 minutes or until the
cranberries are partially cooked.

4. Meanwhile, stir the gelatin into the remaining
hot water until dissolved. While the cranberries
are simmering, stir the gelatin mixture into the
cranberry mixture. Return to a boil. Reduce the
heat and continue to simmer. When cooked, stir
in the vanilla and orange extract.

5. Refrigerate the cranberry mixture until partially set, and then spread it on the prepared marzipan crust. Refrigerate until set, 1 to 2 hours. After the tart is set, cover with plastic wrap. Tart can be made the day before needed, or make the crust the day before and cover and refrigerate. Leftovers will keep for 3 to 4 days.

Preparation Time:
30 minutes

Serves 16

Serving Size:
1/16 cheese-
cake

Lemon Cheesecake

Here's a dessert that's designed for cheesecake lovers. And it's much lower in fat than the traditional version. The crust is made from ground pecans, but you don't need a lot of them to impart the tasty flavor of these nuts. Since the crust is made by spreading a layer of pecans on the bottom of the pan, you will need to carefully spoon the cheesecake mixture over them to make sure they remain in place. Note that I call for a commercial blend of sugar and Splenda, since it gives good results in this recipe.

Nonstick cooking spray

3/4 cup very finely ground pecans (1 cup whole pecans)

1 3/4 cups fat-free cottage cheese

1 cup plain low-fat yogurt

1/2 cup Splenda Sugar Blend for baking or 1 cup Splenda

1/2 cup fat-free liquid egg substitute

2 Tbsp white flour

2 tsp vanilla extract

Zest (grated rind) of one small lemon

4 oz fat-free cream cheese plus 4 oz reduced-fat cream cheese, at room temperature

Exchanges

1 Carbohydrate

1 Fat

Calories 117

Calories from Fat 45

Total Fat 5 g

Saturated Fat 1.4 g

Cholesterol 8 mg

Sodium 197 mg

Total Carbohydrate 11 g

Dietary Fiber 0 g

Sugars 8 g

Protein 7 g

1. Preheat the oven to 350 degrees.

2. Spray a 10-inch springform pan with nonstick cooking spray.

3. Sprinkle the ground pecans evenly over the pan bottom, patting them into place. The crust layer

will be very light and may not entirely cover the bottom of the pan.

4. In a food processor fitted with the plastic blade, process the cottage cheese for 1 minute. Add the yogurt, Splenda Sugar Blend, egg substitute, flour, vanilla, and lemon zest. Process until partially smoothed, about 1 1/2 minutes.

5. Cut the cream cheese into 9 or 10 chunks. One at a time, add the chunks through the feed tube. Process after each addition. Process until smooth—an additional 1 1/2 to 2 minutes.

6. Carefully spoon the mixture over the ground pecans.

7. Bake in the center of the preheated oven for 15 minutes.

8. Lower the oven temperature to 325 degrees and bake for an additional 25 to 35 minutes or until the cheesecake edges have just begun to brown and about an inch of the center jiggles when the pan is lightly shaken. Do not overbake or the cheesecake will crack.

9. Remove to a rack and cool for 20 minutes. Refrigerate at least 6 hours or overnight until cooled. When cooled, cover with plastic wrap.

10. If desired, top with cut fruit.

Dessert Sauce for Fruit

Serves 8

Serving Size:
2 Tbsp

For an easy and elegant sauce for strawberries or mixed fruit, try this sweetened mixture of sour cream and ricotta cheese. The recipe is easy to double if you want to serve it at a party. Because the sauce contains ricotta cheese, be sure to process it for at least a minute and a half so the texture will be smooth.

1 cup nonfat sour cream

1/4 cup nonfat ricotta cheese

3 Tbsp Splenda

1/2 tsp vanilla extract

Exchanges

1 Very Lean Meat

1. In a food processor bowl, combine the sour cream, ricotta, Splenda, and vanilla.

2. Process until smooth, at least 1 1/2 minutes, stopping once and scraping down the sides of the container with a rubber spatula. Transfer to a small bowl and refrigerate, or serve at once on fruit.

Calories 32

Calories from Fat 0

Total Fat 0 g

Saturated Fat 0 g

Cholesterol 5 mg

Sodium 22 mg

Total Carbohydrate
2 g

Dietary Fiber 0 g

Sugars 2 g

Protein 3 g

Greek-Style Quiche

Preparation Time: 15 minutes without crust

Serves 9

Serving Size: 1/9 quiche

There's no need for a crust with this tasty quiche. Simply pour the filling mixture right into the prepared pie plate and bake it.

Nonstick cooking spray
1 1/2 cups frozen cut-leaf spinach
1 cup liquid egg substitute
3/4 cup fat-free ricotta cheese
2 Tbsp white flour
1 1/2 cups shredded fat-free mozzarella cheese
1/2 cup crumbled reduced-fat feta cheese
1 Tbsp olive oil
1 1/2 tsp dried dill weed
1 tsp minced garlic

1. Preheat the oven to 350 degrees. Spray a 9-inch pie plate with nonstick cooking spray and set aside.

2. Place the spinach in a small microwave-safe bowl, cover with wax paper, and microwave on low for 4 or 5 minutes, or until the spinach is thawed. Press any excess water from the spinach.

3. In a large bowl, whisk together the egg substitute, ricotta, and flour. Stir in the mozzarella, feta, olive oil, dill, and garlic. Stir in the spinach.

4. Transfer to the pie plate. Bake for 35 to 40 minutes until set, browned around the edges, and firm in the middle.

Exchanges

1/2 Carbohydrate
2 Very Lean Meat

Calories 105
Calories from Fat 24
Total Fat 3 g
Saturated Fat 0.9 g
Cholesterol 12 mg
Sodium 427 mg
Total Carbohydrate 6 g
Dietary Fiber 1 g
Sugars 2 g
Protein 14 g

Marzipan Candy

*One of my favorite candies is marzipan. So I was
excited to devise this easy, delicious, and sugar-free
method of making it.*

1 6-oz package blanched, slivered almonds
1 cup Splenda
2 Tbsp liquid egg substitute
2 tsp almond extract
1 tsp lemon juice

1. In food processor, process the almonds until
   very finely ground. Turn off the machine and
   add the Splenda, egg substitute, almond extract,
   and lemon juice. Process until the mixture forms
   a ball, or is well combined.

2. Transfer to a 1-quart or similar microwave-safe
   shallow casserole or plastic container. Press the
   marzipan into place. Cover with wax paper and
   microwave for about 4 minutes at 30 percent
   power, until firm but not dry. Cool. With a
   sharp knife, cut into squares.

3. Store tightly covered in the refrigerator. Marzipan will keep for up to 10 days.

Exchanges

1 Fat

Calories 38

Calories from Fat 26

Total Fat 3 g

Saturated Fat 0 g

Cholesterol 0 mg

Sodium 3 mg

Total Carbohydrate
2 g

Dietary Fiber 1 g

Sugars 1 g

Protein 1 g

Marzipan Crust

Preparation Time: 10 minutes

Serves 8

Serving Size: 1/8 crust

I use this wonderful crust for both my fruit tart and my cranberry-orange tart.

1 6-oz package blanched, slivered almonds
1/4 cup liquid egg substitute
1/3 cup Splenda
2 Tbsp warm water
1 tsp almond extract

1. In a food processor, process the almonds until they are very finely ground.

2. Turn off the machine and add the egg substitute, Splenda, water, and almond extract. Process until well combined.

3. Transfer to a 9- or 10-inch microwave-safe dinner plate. Pat and shape into a circle with a slight raised area at the edge. Cover with wax paper and microwave on high power for about 2 minutes or until the crust is somewhat firm. If the crust has risen from center of plate, press it back into place.

4. Continue to microwave, covered with wax paper, in 30-second increments, until the crust is almost dry in the center, about 1 to 2 more minutes. Set the plate on a wire rack to cool slightly.

Exchanges

1/2 Carbohydrate

2 Fat

Calories 137

Calories from Fat 102

Total Fat 11 g

Saturated Fat 0.9 g

Cholesterol 0 mg

Sodium 15 mg

Total Carbohydrate 5 g

Dietary Fiber 3 g

Sugars 2 g

Protein 5

Easy Pastry Crust

Preparation Time:
20 minutes

Serves 8

Serving Size:
1/8 pie

I've always considered traditional pie crust one of the least nutritious foods you could eat, since it's sky-high in both fat and carb. Here's one that's better for you. There's relatively little fat and some protein from the soy flour, which is available at health-food stores. Another plus is that the crust is relatively thin, especially when made in a deep-dish pie plate. This recipe makes crust for a regular or deep-dish 9-inch pie.

If you hate rolling out pie crust the way I do, you'll find this one easy to make, because you mix it right in the pie plate and then press it into place. When I make the crust, I distribute most of the mixture over the bottom and sides of the plate and then press the sides into place first, using my thumb to hold the upper edge in place as I work. When the sides are in place, I smooth out the bottom of the crust. Finally, I press the crust down around the edges of the plate with a fork to make an attractive edge.

Exchanges

1 Starch

1 1/2 Fat

Calories 128

Calories from Fat 72

Total Fat 8 g

Saturated Fat 1 g

Cholesterol 0 mg

Sodium 76 mg

Total Carbohydrate 11 g

Dietary Fiber 1 g

Sugars 2 g

Protein 3 g

3/4 cup white flour

1/2 cup soy flour

1/4 tsp salt

1/4 cup canola oil

2 Tbsp plus 2 tsp fat-free milk (or a little more if necessary)

1. In a 9-inch pie plate or deep-dish pie plate, carefully stir together the flours and salt with a fork.

2. In a 1-cup measure, beat together the oil and milk with a fork, until the milk is completely incorporated.

3. Gradually add the oil mixture to the flours, stirring with a spoon as you pour it in. Use your fingers to finish working the liquid into the dry ingredients. If the mixture will not hold together, add a few more drops of milk to make it workable. But do not over-moisten the pastry.

4. When the ingredients are well blended, press the mixture into place in the pie plate with your fingers, working it out evenly over the sides and bottom and over the top edge. Crimp the edge with the tines of a fork.

5. Lightly cover with plastic wrap and allow to rest at room temperature for 10 to 20 minutes while you prepare the filling ingredients.

6. Follow the recipe directions for the specific pie.

Preparation Time:
12 minutes

Serves 7

Serving Size:
1 cup

Mulled "Cider"

I've always loved the taste of hot mulled cider. This hot winter drink tastes a lot like traditional mulled cider, but has fewer calories. It's easy to double the recipe if you want to serve a large pot of this flavorful hot punch.

6 cups hot decaffeinated or caffeinated tea

1 cup orange juice

2 Tbsp lemon juice

3/4 cup Splenda, or to taste

1/2 tsp vanilla

1/4 tsp orange extract

1 cinnamon stick

6 whole cloves

1. Combine all the ingredients in a large saucepan. Bring to a simmer. Simmer for 20 minutes to allow the spices to permeate the liquid.

2. Ladle into mugs. Leftovers will keep in the refrigerator for 2 to 3 days. Rewarm in the microwave.

Exchanges

1/2 Carbohydrate

Calories 30

Calories from Fat 1

Total Fat 0 g

Saturated Fat 0 g

Cholesterol 0 mg

Sodium 7 mg

Total Carbohydrate
7 g

Dietary Fiber 0 g

Sugars 6 g

Protein 0 g

Peanut Butter and Marmalade Sandwich

This is one of my favorite snack recipes, because it has the taste of peanut butter and marmalade without any extra sugar.

1 Tbsp natural (nonhydrogenated, no-sugar) peanut butter
1/2 tsp Splenda, or to taste
1/8 tsp orange extract
1 slice low-carb or regular whole-wheat bread
1 medium apple, sliced

1. In a small bowl, blend the peanut butter, Splenda, and orange extract together with a fork.

2. Spread on whole-wheat bread. Serve sandwich with the apple.

Exchanges

1 1/2 Starch

1 Fruit

1 High-Fat Meat

Calories 294

Calories from Fat 101

Total Fat 11 g

Saturated Fat 2.0 g

Cholesterol 0 mg

Sodium 311 mg

Total Carbohydrate 40 g

Dietary Fiber 10 g

Sugars 15 g

Protein 13 g

Serves 1

Serving Size:
1 cup

Curried Peanut Soup

Quick, easy, and tangy, this soup is great for a cold winter day. I prefer to make it with peanut butter that hasn't been refrigerated. If you have only refrigerated peanut butter, you will need to bring it to room temperature in the microwave before making the soup.

2 Tbsp fat-free sour cream

1 Tbsp natural peanut butter, at room temperature

1/2 tsp mild curry powder, or to taste

1 cup reduced-sodium chicken broth

1. In a small bowl, whisk together the sour cream, peanut butter, and curry powder until smooth.

2. Gradually whisk in the chicken broth until well combined.

3. Microwave for 1 minute.

4. Pour into a mug.

Exchanges

1 High-Fat Meat

1/2 Carbohydrate

Calories 138

Calories from Fat 73

Total Fat 8 g

Saturated Fat 1 g

Cholesterol 2 mg

Sodium 595 mg

Total Carbohydrate 9 g

Dietary Fiber 1 g

Sugars 4 g

Protein 7 g

Pecan Pie Crust

Preparation Time:
20 minutes

Serves 8

Serving Size:
1/8 crust

This richly flavored crust makes a nice change from a graham cracker crust. The recipe makes crust for a 9-inch pie.

1 1/4 cups very finely ground pecans
2 Tbsp Splenda
2 Tbsp melted reduced-fat margarine or butter

1. Preheat the oven to 400 degrees.

2. In a small bowl, mix together the pecans and Splenda. Stir in the butter. Moisten your fingers with water and press the mixture firmly against the bottom and sides of the pie plate. Quickly press a base of crust into the flat portion of the plate. Then work some of the mixture up the sides of the plate. Finally, return to the middle and smooth out the crust into a thin layer. If the crust sticks to your fingers, moisten them again. If the crust is for an unbaked pie filling, bake the crust until it is lightly browned, about 6 to 8 minutes.

Exchanges
2 1/2 Fat

Calories 118

Total Fat 12 g

Saturated Fat 1 g

Calories from Fat 110

Cholesterol 0 mg

Sodium 19 mg

Total Carbohydrate
2 g

Dietary Fiber 1 g

Sugars 1 g

Protein 1 g

Spiced Pecans

Here's one of my favorite ways to give pecans a sweet and spicy flavor boost.

1/2 Tbsp low-fat buttery spread
1/2 tsp pumpkin pie spice
1 cup pecan halves
1/2 Tbsp sugar-free pancake syrup
1/2 tsp vanilla extract

1. In a medium-sized skillet, melt the spread over medium heat. Stir in the pumpkin pie spice. Add the pecans and cook, stirring, over medium heat for 5 minutes, until the nuts are sautéed and the flavors are blended.

2. Remove from the heat. Add the syrup and vanilla and stir well to combine.

3. Transfer the nuts to a plate, spreading them out. Allow to cool. Serve at once, or store in a tightly closed container in the refrigerator. The nuts will keep for several weeks.

Exchanges

1 1/2 Fat

Calories 73

Calories from Fat 68

Total Fat 8 g

Saturated Fat 0.7 g

Cholesterol 0 mg

Sodium 5 mg

Total Carbohydrate
1 g

Dietary Fiber 1 g

Sugars 0 g

Protein 1 g

Salmon Spread

Preparation Time:
15 minutes

Serves 16

Serving Size:
1 Tbsp

Here's a tasty spread you can use as an appetizer or a snack.

1 6-oz can boneless, skinless salmon, drained
3 oz reduced-fat cream cheese cut into 3 or 4
    pieces
3 Tbsp chopped pecans
1 tsp lemon juice
1 tsp instant minced onion
1/4 tsp dried dill weed
1 tsp prepared white horseradish
1/8 tsp salt, or to taste
2 to 3 drops hot pepper sauce
1/4 cup finely chopped celery

1. In a food processor container, combine the
   salmon, cream cheese, pecans, lemon juice,
   onion, dill, horseradish, salt, and hot pepper
   sauce. Process until almost completely smooth.
   Stir in the celery.

2. Transfer to a small serving bowl. Serve with
   crackers or celery sticks. Serve at once, or cover
   and refrigerate. The spread will keep in the
   refrigerator for 4 or 5 days.

Exchanges
1 Fat

Calories 37
Calories from Fat 25
Total Fat 3 g
Saturated Fat 1.0 g
Cholesterol 8 mg
Sodium 90 mg
Total Carbohydrate
    1 g
Dietary Fiber 0 g
Sugars 0 g
Protein 2 g

Serves 20

Serving Size:
1/20
cheesecake

Summer Cheesecake

Here's an easy summer cheesecake with a wonderful flavor. One of the ingredients is fat-free evaporated milk. When chilled to a very cold temperature, it can be whipped just like cream. If you want to be sure the milk is cold enough, chill it until ice crystals begin to form around the edges.

Nonstick cooking spray

1 3/4 cups finely ground graham cracker crumbs, divided

1 12-oz can fat-free evaporated milk, divided

2 packets unflavored gelatin

1 cup boiling water

1/4 cup lemon juice

4 oz fat-free plus 4 oz reduced-fat cream cheese, cut into chunks

1/2 cup Splenda Sugar Blend or 1 cup Splenda

1 tsp vanilla

Exchanges

1 Carbohydrate

1/2 Fat

Calories 95

Calories from Fat 19

Total Fat 2 g

Saturated Fat 0.9 g

Cholesterol 5 mg

Sodium 143 mg

Total Carbohydrate 15 g

Dietary Fiber 0 g

Sugars 9 g

Protein 4 g

1. Spray a 9- by 13-inch pan with nonstick cooking spray. Sprinkle 1 1/2 cups graham cracker crumbs evenly over the pan bottom and press them firmly against bottom of pan.

2. Pour 1/4 cup of the evaporated milk into a food processor bowl fitted with the plastic blade and set aside. Pour the remaining milk into a mixing bowl (preferably metal) and put into the freezer.

3. In a measuring cup, sprinkle the gelatin over the boiling water. Stir until the gelatin is dissolved, about 1 or 2 minutes. Add the lemon juice. Reserve.

4. To the food processor bowl, add the cream cheese, Splenda Sugar Blend, and vanilla. Process until smooth, about 2 minutes. Pour in the gelatin mixture through the feed tube. Process until well combined.

5. When the remaining evaporated milk is very cold, beat on high speed with an electric mixer until lightly whipped, about a minute and a half. Reduce the speed to medium. With the mixer running, beat in the cream cheese mixture.

6. Spoon the mixture into the prepared crust and sprinkle with the remaining crumbs. Refrigerate until set, about 2 hours. Cover. The cheesecake will keep in the refrigerator for 3 to 4 days.

Preparation Time:
25 minutes

Serves 9

Serving Size:
1/9 pie or
custard

Sweet Potato Pie

This recipe is a little more work than some. But it's worth it, because sweet potatoes are so good for you and because the pie tastes so delicious. I use fresh sweet potatoes and microwave them while I'm preparing the other ingredients. Two cups is about two large sweet potatoes.

To make this recipe easier, you can turn it into a custard by leaving off the crust. For both the custard and the pie, I use a 9-inch deep-dish pie plate.

Nonstick cooking spray
1 Easy Pastry Crust (see recipe, p. 206)
1/2 cup liquid egg substitute
1 12-oz can evaporated fat-free milk
1 tsp vanilla extract
2 cups cooked, mashed sweet potato
2/3 cup Splenda
2 tsp pumpkin pie spice
1/2 tsp ground ginger

Exchanges (with crust)

1 1/2 Fat

2 Carbohydrate

Calories 209

Calories from Fat 65

Total Fat 7 g

Saturated Fat 1 g

Cholesterol 0 mg

Sodium 151 mg

Total Carbohydrate
28 g

Dietary Fiber 2 g

Sugars 12 g

Protein 8 g

1. If making a pie, prepare the pastry crust at least 20 minutes before needed. If making a custard, spray the pie plate with nonstick spray and set aside. Preheat the oven to 350 degrees.

2. In a 2-cup measure or similar small bowl, combine the egg substitute, milk, and vanilla. Set aside.

3. Place the sweet potatoes in a mixer bowl and beat slightly at low speed to smooth. Add the Splenda, pumpkin pie spice, ginger, and about 1/2 cup of the milk mixture, continuing to beat at medium speed. When incorporated, slowly beat in the remaining milk mixture, stopping and scraping the sides and bottom of the bowl as necessary, beating for about 4 or 5 minutes until the mixture is smooth.

4. Pour the filling into the pie plate and bake in the center of the oven for 42 to 45 minutes or until set and browned around the edges. A toothpick inserted in the center should come out clean.

Exchanges (without crust)

1 Carbohydrate

Calories 95

Calories from Fat 2

Total Fat 0 g

Saturated Fat 0 g

Cholesterol 0 mg

Sodium 84 mg

Total Carbohydrate 18 g

Dietary Fiber 1 g

Sugars 11 g

Protein 5 g

Serves 2

Serving Size:
1/2 cup

Quick Sweet Potato Snacks

Try this easy and very tasty way to enjoy a sweet potato. Microwave cooking makes preparation a snap.

1 medium sweet potato
1 tsp Splenda
1 tsp olive oil
1/2 tsp orange extract
1/4 tsp pumpkin pie spice
2 Tbsp chopped pecans or walnuts

1. Lay the sweet potato on a plate. Pierce the potato in several places with a knife or a fork. Microwave on high power for about 7 minutes or until cooked through.

2. Cut the sweet potato in half. Scoop out the flesh onto a medium-sized plate. Mash with a fork.

3. Mash in the Splenda, oil, orange extract, and pumpkin pie spice. Stir in the nuts. Leftovers can be covered, refrigerated, and reheated in the microwave.

Exchanges
1 Starch
1 1/2 Fat

Calories 133

Calories from Fat 68

Total Fat 8 g

Saturated Fat 1 g

Cholesterol 0 mg

Sodium 6 mg

Total Carbohydrate 15 g

Dietary Fiber 2 g

Sugars 7 g

Protein 2 g

Teriyaki Chicken Bites

Preparation Time:
15 minutes

Serves 6

Serving Size:
4 pieces

These tasty chicken bites are great party food. You can make them in the broiler, but they cook much more quickly in a George Foreman grill.

3 Tbsp lite soy sauce

2 Tbsp peanut oil

1 tsp rice vinegar or white vinegar

1 tsp Splenda

1/2 tsp ground ginger

1 tsp minced garlic

1 lb boneless, skinless chicken breast

1. In a large bowl or ceramic casserole, mix together the soy sauce, oil, vinegar, Splenda, ginger, and garlic.

2. With a sharp knife, cut the chicken into bite-sized pieces.

3. Put the chicken into the bowl with the marinade. Stir to coat. Cover and refrigerate for 2 to 3 hours or up to 12 hours, stirring occasionally.

4. If broiling, transfer the chicken and marinade to a 9 1/2- by 13-inch baking pan. Broil about 4 inches from the heat, turning chicken and basting occasionally with the sauce, for 17 to 20 minutes until the chicken pieces are cooked through and begin to brown. If using a George Foreman grill, grill for about 5 to 6 minutes. Serve warm with toothpicks. Chicken can be cooked ahead and reheated in the broiler or microwave.

Exchanges
2 Lean Meat

Calories 119
Calories from Fat 44
Total Fat 5 g
Saturated Fat 1 g
Cholesterol 46 mg
Sodium 242 mg
Total Carbohydrate
1 g
Dietary Fiber 0 g
Sugars 1 g
Protein 17 g

Serves 2

Serving Size:
scant 1 cup

Tomato Soup with a Difference

This recipe may look unusual, but the peanut butter added to this tomato soup gives it a very pleasing flavor. I use a large saucepan to give myself ample room for whisking.

2 Tbsp natural peanut butter, at room temperature

1 cup reduced-sodium or regular chicken broth

1/2 cup low-sodium or regular tomato sauce

1/4 cup reduced-fat (2%) milk

Dash onion powder

2–3 drops hot pepper sauce

Exchanges

1 High-Fat Meat

1/2 Carbohydrate

Calories 135

Calories from Fat 77

Total Fat 9 g

Saturated Fat 1 g

Cholesterol 2 mg

Sodium 343 mg

Total Carbohydrate 9 g

Dietary Fiber 2 g

Sugars 6 g

Protein 6 g

1. Place the peanut butter in a large saucepan. Warm over medium-low heat. Slowly whisk in 1/3 of the chicken broth at a time, whisking well after each addition, until blended. If the peanut butter will not combine, transfer to a blender. Blend on high speed for about 1 minute or until smooth before returning the mixture to the pan.

2. Add the tomato sauce, milk, onion powder, and hot pepper sauce. Heat until warmed.

3. Pour into two mugs and serve.

Mexican Tuna Dip

Preparation Time:
10 minutes

Serves 10

Serving Size:
2 Tbsp

In La Paz, Mexico, while you sit in a restaurant and contemplate the sea and palm trees, you can enjoy an interesting variation on the standard chips and dip appetizer. Instead of salsa, the waiter is likely to set out a creamy dip that's enlivened with canned tuna. Here's my version. At home, I serve this dip with celery sticks, broccoli, and cauliflower as well as fat-free baked corn chips.

1/2 cup reduced-fat mayonnaise

1/4 cup reduced-fat sour cream

3 Tbsp mild or medium salsa

2 tsp Splenda

2 tsp cider vinegar

1 6-oz can albacore tuna, drained and flaked

1. Mix together the mayonnaise, sour cream, and salsa. Stir in the Splenda and vinegar. Stir in the tuna. Serve at once or refrigerate. Dip will keep in the refrigerator for 2 to 3 days.

2. Serve with fat-free tortilla chips or vegetables. For a larger snack portion, spread 3 Tbsp on a piece of whole-wheat bread.

Exchanges

1 Very Lean Meat

1 Fat

Calories 66

Calories from Fat 42

Total Fat 5 g

Saturated Fat 1 g

Cholesterol 10 mg

Sodium 164 mg

Total Carbohydrate 2 g

Dietary Fiber 0 g

Sugars 0 g

Protein 4 g

Alphabetical Index

Subject Index

Beans *(continued)*
Chickpea and Sun-Dried Tomato
  Spread, 14
Con Queso Bean Dip, 161
Luscious Limas, 109
Marinated Green Beans, 113
Pasta, Bean, and Salmon Salad, 123
Red, White, and Green Bean Dip,
  191
Salsa Bean Dip, 192
Three-Bean Snack, 129

Beef
Cocktail Meatballs, 82
Hawaiian Meatballs, 84

Beverages
Banana-Strawberry Shake, 47
Mango Lassi, 46
Mulled "Cider," 208
Strawberry-Peach Cooler, 45

Blueberries
Blueberry Muffins, 186
Red, White, and Blue Fruit Tart,
  197

Cabbage
Cabbage and Carrot Slaw, 116
Cabbage and Peanut Slaw, 196

Carrots
Cabbage and Carrot Slaw, 116
Carrot-Raisin Salad, 119
Pineapple-Carrot Muffins, 182

Celery
Celery Man, 136
Stuffed Celery Sticks, 114

Cheese
Apples and Cheese, 54
Blue Cheese Spread, 193

Cottage Cheese with Dill and
  Onion, 5
Easy Cheese Popcorn, 50
Easy Cheese Sauce, 103
Feta-Stuffed New Potatoes, 96
Ham and Cheese Puffs, 68
Mini Spinach and Cheese Calzone,
  66
Spinach, Red Onion, and Cheese
  Pizza, 60

Cherries
Cherry Tarts, 173

Chicken
Barbecued Chicken Pizza, 64
Italian Chicken Nuggets, 80
Middle Eastern–Style Chicken, 86
Teriyaki Chicken Bites, 219

Chickpeas
Chickpea and Sun-Dried Tomato
  Spread, 14
Falafel, 28
Israeli Chickpeas, 107

Corn
Bean and Corn Con Carne Soup,
  78
Bean, Corn, and Rice Salad, 117
Easy Corn Relish, 44

Desserts
Apple Betty, 168
Apple-Cranberry Turnovers, 189
Apple Crisp, 185
Apple Scone Cake, 164
Apricot Kuchen, 176
Banana Pops, 155
Caramel Apples, 146
Cherry Tarts, 173
Cinnamon Triangles, 153
Cranberry-Orange Tart, 198

Salmon Salad, 11
Spanish Rice Salad, 121
Tabouli, 131
Three-Bean Snack, 129
Tuna Salad, 12
Turkey Bulgur Salad, 132
Turkey Salad with Apples and
    Almonds, 133

Salmon
Pasta, Bean, and Salmon Salad, 123
Salmon Mousse, 92
Salmon Salad, 11
Salmon Spread, 213

Sandwiches
At the Zoo, 150
Bread Puzzle, 149
Egg 'n' Muffin, 22
Egg 'n' Muffin, Italian Style, 24
Egg 'n' Muffin, Mexican Style, 23
Egg Salad Sandwich, 38
Eggplant Mini-Pita Pocket
    Sandwiches, 30
Falafel, 28
Grilled Portobello Mushroom
    Sandwich, 25
Middle Eastern Sandwich, 27
Pan-Grilled Vegetable Wrap, 36
Peanut Butter and Marmalade
    Sandwich, 209
Pepper and Onion Quesadilla, 32
Quick Fajitas, 26
Quick Turkey Salad Sandwich, 39
Tuna Melts, 33
Turkey and Tomato Wrap, 34
Vegetable Wrap, 35

Sauces
Dessert Sauce for Fruit, 202
Easy Cheese Sauce, 103
Mixed Herb Pesto, 19
Sun-Dried Tomato Pesto, 20

Tangy Mustard Sauce, 159
Thousand Island Dressing, 8

Shrimp
Artichoke and Shrimp Spread, 4
Artichoke, Shrimp, and Roasted
    Red Pepper Pizza, 62
Shrimp Remoulade, 98

Soup
Bean and Corn Con Carne Soup, 78
Bean and Pasta Soup with Sausage,
    77
Curried Peanut Soup, 210
Tomato Soup with a Difference, 220
West African Sweet Potato–Peanut
    Soup, 79

Spinach
Mini Spinach and Cheese Calzone,
    66
Spinach, Red Onion, and Cheese
    Pizza, 60

Strawberries
Banana-Strawberry Shake, 47
Red, White, and Blue Fruit Tart, 197
Strawberry-Peach Cooler, 45

Stuffing
Fruit Stuffing Pronto, 163
Stuffing Pronto, 162

Sweet Potatoes
Quick Sweet Potato Snacks, 218
Sweet Potato Pie, 216
Sweet Potatoes Supreme, 160
West African Sweet Potato–Peanut
    Soup, 79

Tomatoes
Chickpea and Sun-Dried Tomato
    Spread, 14

Other Titles Available from Small Steps Press

What to Eat When You're Eating Out
By Hope S. Warshaw, MMSc, RD
This comprehensive book provides complete nutrition information for more than 5,000 menu items from more than 60 restaurants, along with strategies for choosing healthier foods when eating out.
Order #4723-01
$9.95 US

The Healthy Lunchbox: How to Plan, Prepare, and Pack Stress-Free Meals Kids Will Love
By Marie McClendon, MEd, and Cristy Shauck
Do your kids groan when they look inside their lunchboxes? Do the nutritious meals you pack return home uneaten? Are you having trouble finding suitable and tasty recipes for your child with special eating needs? This unique guide is filled with helpful tips, tricks, and techniques for preparing quick and easy healthy meals.
Order #5013-01
$12.95 US

The Ultimate Calorie, Carb, and Fat Gram Counter
By Lea Ann Holzmeister, RD, CDE
If you want to lose weight or just keep track of how much fat or how many carbs you're eating, let this handy reference be your guide. Packed with information, this book features nutrient counts for more than 7,000 fresh, packaged, and restaurant foods.
Order #4724-01
$9.95 US

Disease Prevention Cookbook
By Clara Schneider, MS, RD, RN, LD, CDE
This innovative cookbook is filled with delicious recipes and tools designed to help you prevent some of the most prevalent diseases in our society, including diabetes, heart disease, stroke, and cancer.
Order #4651-01
$14.95 US

To order these and other great Small Steps Press titles, call 1-800-232-6733 or visit http://store.diabetes.org. Small Steps Press titles are also available in bookstores nationwide.